YOGA

FOR A HAPPY BACK

YOGA

FOR A HAPPY BACK

A Teacher's Guide to
Spinal Health through
Yoga Therapy

RACHEL
KRENTZMAN PT, E-RYT
Foreword by Aadil Palkhivala

SINGING
DRAGON

LONDON AND PHILADELPHIA

First published in 2016
by Singing Dragon
an imprint of Jessica Kingsley Publishers
73 Collier Street
London N1 9BE, UK
and
400 Market Street, Suite 400
Philadelphia, PA 19106, USA

www.singingdragon.com

Library of Congress Cataloging in Publication Data
Names: Krentzman, Rachel.
Title: Yoga for a happy back : a teacher's guide to spinal health through
yoga therapy / Rachel Krentzman ; foreword by Aadil Palkhivala.
Description: London ; Philadelphia : Singing Dragon, 2016. | Includes
bibliographical references and index.
Identifiers: LCCN 2015041437 | ISBN 9781848192713 (alk. paper)
Subjects: LCSH: Back--Care and hygiene--Popular works. | Back
exercises--Popular works. | Backache--Exercise therapy--Popular works. |
Backache--Alternative treatment--Popular works. | Yoga--Therapeutic
use--Popular works.
Classification: LCC RD768 .K74 2016 | DDC 613.7/046--dc23 LC
record available at http://lccn.loc.gov/2015041437

British Library Cataloguing in Publication Data
A CIP catalogue record for this book is available from the British Library

ISBN 978 1 84819 271 3
eISBN 978 0 85701 253 1

Printed and bound in Great Britain

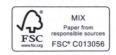

To my teachers

Of yoga and life—Aadil Palkhivala, Aman Keays, and Amy Caldwell
Of persistence and faith—Marc Zegans and Anne Marie Welsh
Of family and forgiveness—Tova, Adeena, Daniel, and Ariella Krentzman
Of unconditional love—my sons, Jake and Noam
Of sanctuary and surrender—the ocean and the sea

Contents

Part I: Principles and Practices of Yoga for a Happy Back

Part II: Teaching Yoga for a Happy Back

Foreword

"Don't worry; I've got your back."

"The wall needs strong backing."

"When I present my case, will you back me up?"

"If I cannot teach tonight, will you be my backup?"

In our language itself, we use the word *back* to mean support. We have learned to believe that our back is, indeed, that which reinforces us, that which buttresses us, that which holds us up.

Other phrases—"Back in the good old days," or "In the back of my mind, I believe…," or "Before you hire him, do a background check," or "Do you have the back issues of the magazine?," or "One day you will look back and be glad you did this"—remind us that in our language the word *back* also equates with the past. Our back, therefore, must hold the joy and the sorrow, the strength and the fear, the power and the insecurity of our yesteryears.

Thus our mind believes that "back" represents *both* support and the past. So, when I sense the familiarity of being unsupported, when I feel out-of-control or perceive fear, this thought-sense with its entourage of emotions floods my defenseless subconscious mind.

Since no one can show where the mind ends and the body begins, what happens in my mind must be reflected and manifested in my body. What I feel determines how my body responds. If I feel unsupported, unstable, or burdened by the past, my back must show it to me by giving me discomfort and pain.

It is impossible to facilitate true and long-term healing in my body or the body of my students by merely doing some stretching exercises. The mind, the body, and the emotions must all be addressed. Having suffered intense back pain originating from two herniated discs and severe sacroiliac misalignment, I know from personal experience that true healing of the back must be a multi-pronged process. Using asana and specialty traction devices which I designed, I was able to ease my lower back pain, yet it would spring up unashamedly and humiliate me when I was least expecting it! Only after dealing with the entire mind–body–emotion–spirit continuum did my intense lower back pain begin to fade into memory. It's the scientific magic of Purna Yoga,™ which includes Savitri's Heartfull™ Meditation, Philosophy, and Lifestyle. Savitri and I have successfully treated thousands of students with lower back pain. This is why, in the work that Rachel Krentzman presents in this book, you will learn to address more than the mere symptoms in your body. After all, are we not far more than merely flesh and bones?

As a teacher of yoga it is your duty to help your students by addressing them as whole human beings, not solely as a body. As a student of yoga it is to your advantage to find a teacher who has had extensive training in our Purna Yoga system and continues ongoing study; Rachel Krentzman is such a teacher. Be willing to look into your past to understand your current condition. Of course, carefully address your body, since that is where the pain is manifesting itself now. Explore and understand the physiology of your lower back so that you can give your back precise and prudent physical amelioration. Yet, do not ignore your mind or your history. As George Eliot wrote:

Our deeds still travel with us from afar,

And what we have been makes us what we are.

Rachel has been my student for many years and has more than 2000 hours of Purna Yoga teacher training and additional therapeutic teacher training, making her one of the most qualified yoga teachers anywhere. I request that you read this book carefully, imbibe its contents, and practice the techniques. One day you will look back and be glad you did.

May great teachers, teachers who *live* their yoga, be your outer guides. May the light of your Spirit be your inner guide.

May Purna Yoga give you more than pain relief. May it help you to explore yourself, find yourself, love yourself.

Aadil Palkhivala
Yoga-Asana Master, Co-founder of Purna Yoga, Attorney at Law

Acknowledgments

First, I would like to offer boundless thanks to all of my yoga teachers who have helped shape my practice and my life: Aadil Palkhivala, Judith Hanson Lasater, Aman and Sunny Keays, Jo Zukovich, Roger Cole, Matthew Taylor, and Prasad Ragnekar.

To all the studio owners who gave me the opportunity to teach and work tirelessly to keep yoga accessible to everyone: Gerhard and Alexandra Gessner from Prana Yoga Center, Amy and Michael Caldwell from Yoga One, and Brad and Cindy Bennett from Ginseng Yoga.

To all my students, patients, and friends without whom I would have no stories to tell. There are too many to thank individually, but here are a few: Aparna Bharati, Sharon Roy, Denise Rhodes, Anna Holden, Sofie Bundy, Rosemary Caddy, Mike St. John, Todd Sykes, Nauder Motamedi, and Kimberley Bell.

To my trusty assistants over the years: Jaimie Perkunas, Shawnee Thornton Hardy, Lauren Bosworth, Christine Carr, Jason Cull, and Alex Van Frank.

To the core staff at Embody Physical Therapy & Yoga for their commitment and dedication and to holding down the fort while I wrote this book: Nicole Mullins, Amanda Cravinho, Alison McLean, and Jennifer Chang.

To Dr. Melanie Fiorella, Lauray MacElhern, and Renee Lewis and the staff at the UCSD Center for Integrative Medicine.

To Dr. Loren Fishman for his encouragement and his evidence-based contributions to the yoga therapy field, and to John Kepner and the International Association of Yoga Therapists which he directs.

To Laura Carr for all her support.

To my talented and amazing photographer Tim Hardy and my artist extraordinaire Lior Hikrey.

Immense gratitude to my editor and dear friend, Anne Marie Welsh, for her invaluable input into this project.

And finally to my creative business coach, Marc Zegans, who helped me see that anything is possible.

Introduction

**We spend our life fishing
only to realize it is not fish we are after.**
Henry David Thoreau

Every Wednesday I swim in the ocean. I created this ritual more than four years ago. After dropping my son off at school, I head straight to La Jolla Cove and brave the always chilly entrance to the mile-long swim to the buoys. And every year on my birthday, I swim the two-mile cove route to La Jolla Shores and enjoy a birthday brunch with an ocean view. I rarely miss a week unless it has been raining or the swell is too big. I am there, in fog or sunshine, wending my way through the kelp and the unknown.

This cove is a sacred place for me. I left my wedding band near the quarter-mile buoy, knowing the ocean would receive it and hold it for me. I visit it every now and then and use the time out there to pay homage to the dreams I had and the love I was searching for. Sometimes I cry, sometimes I pray, and other times I just swim by and glance back. When I emerge from the ocean, refreshed and humbled, I shower off and go teach my 10 a.m. yoga class. My students are accustomed to me running in with sandy feet and an occasional strand of seaweed in my salty hair. They know it will be a good class if I swam. Swimming in the cove gives me the clarity and focus that I have only otherwise found with a regular yoga practice. It helps me to be fully present and aware and feeds my soul.

Being out in the ocean is a stark reminder of how vulnerable we truly are. I usually swim with a partner for safety and to ease some of the fears of the unknown world below. If my friends cannot make it, I go anyway, but find my mind an interesting beast to tame. I work on constantly redirecting my thoughts away from images from the *Jaws* novel I snuck from my parents' bookshelf and read when I was a child. I just keep my eye on the quarter-mile buoy and swim towards it with certainty that once I reach it, I am safe and protected.

As I swam out towards my buoy on one particular Wednesday, an uneasy feeling came over me. I suddenly and unexpectedly became aware of the illusion my mind had created. I had always seen the buoy as a destination, an island that would save me from anything out there if I could just touch it. The knowledge that it was there gave me direction and a sense of peace. However, when I reached the buoy that day, it hit me that the safety I felt was false. I had created it to feel some sense of control over my environment, but the truth was I was still out at sea and at the mercy of its depths.

We all have our buoys, our illusions that we cling to for safety and security. We learn this at a young age, as we are wired for survival. For some, that buoy is money and a nice home; for others it is family or a significant other, a career, or expertise in a field. We cling to ideas of who we are or who we need to be to feel all right in this world, for this world is like the ocean—vast, expansive, and unpredictable. It can be beautiful and peaceful and, in an instant, become turbulent and hostile.

This "clinging" often manifests as physical tension in the muscles, tissues, and joints. When we are gripping in our minds, we will translate that sense of "holding on for dear life" to our bodies as well. The more we try to control life, the more we tense up. The more we can let go and trust, the more we unwind.

I have spent most of my life trying to control things around me to give me a sense of safety. During my childhood, I did not receive validation for who I really was as an individual, but instead was expected to obey rigid rules of right and wrong. I was the daughter of a strict and distant rabbi, and a child born while another one was dying. I felt that if I won the approval of others, did well, excelled, kept in shape, married a good man, had children, and found a respectable job, my fears would ease. Yet, even though I had achieved most of my goals at a relatively young age, an emptiness inside persisted. I was a closet over-achiever: calm and collected on the outside, a bundle of nerves on the inside. Maintaining constant perfection took a lot of hard work, and even when I achieved excellence, the satisfaction did not last long. There was always another mountain to climb.

Then, I herniated a disc.

It happened during a yoga class after being adjusted in a deep forward bend. I felt shooting pains down my right leg, followed by tingling and numbness with paralysis of my right foot. I knew exactly what level of my spine was affected and what was happening, but could not do anything about it. I spent the next week sleeping on the floor, which gave me plenty of time to think about how this had happened.

I had graduated from physical therapy school in Montreal eight years before, in 1996. My student idealism was quickly stifled two years later when I began working within the healthcare system in the US. I felt limited within that system in my ability to truly heal any one patient. Of course I was able to help, but the system made it difficult to see the same patient twice and allowed approximately 15 to 20 minutes at most with a patient, which was barely time enough to scratch the surface of the patient's condition. We had to log our productivity and were penalized if we did not have enough "billable" hours, a demand which made me feel like I was running around trying to fill time. It was hard to be truly present with any patient.

At the same time, I had begun to experience significant pain and tension in my upper back and shoulder blade area. I had been diagnosed with scoliosis at age 16, but never received any treatment, since the curve was only about 10°. However, all the forward bending and lifting of patients was now taking its toll on my body.

Then, in 1999 and thanks to my sister, I found yoga. I began practicing regularly and started to notice that the pain in my back disappeared. I had more energy overall and felt compelled to eat more healthily. I became more sensitive to the needs of my body. Having had a strong background in anatomy, I was able to see the benefits of the asanas (postures) from the inside out. I began to wonder if I could use these postures in my practice of physical therapy.

After a good deal of research, I found a course offered in Rye, New York, by my now good friend and colleague Matt Taylor. I attended his conference and began using these blended techniques with some patients in an outpatient clinic when I had the chance. Sometimes I had to sneak away with patients so that I could spend more time with them. Ultimately, these clients not only recovered and had a great physiotherapy experience, but they also had tools they needed to practice on their own. Shortly afterwards, I decided to leave the constraints of the clinic and went off to start my own practice out of my garage in Ocean Beach, California.

As I lay there in agony after the injury, what was most difficult for me to understand as I reviewed my choices was why I would have injured myself doing yoga. After all, I had moved away from a rigid medical system toward a more holistic approach to treating patients. But through self-inquiry and self-observation, I realized that it was *how* I practiced the asanas that made all the difference. I was approaching my practice with the same aggression with which I approached my life. Too much effort, not enough ease. I was moving quickly through poses without paying close attention; I focused on how the posture looked, not how it felt. A sense of competitiveness, of having to be the "best," caused me to go more deeply into poses when I should have backed off and focused on strength and stability. Since my lower back is the flexible part of my spine, it took all the wear and tear.

After my week of suffering and self-examination on the floor, I finally had an MRI scan that showed a complete herniation at L5–S1. My doctor took one look at the MRI report and told me that I would have to modify my activities for the rest of my life. "Thank you very much," I said. Then I hung up the phone and never went back to her. At that moment, I began to use yoga and physical therapy to heal myself.

Slowly, my yoga practice deepened and my pain subsided. Two years after the injury, I met the man who would become my teacher, Aadil Palkhivala, at a conference in San Francisco. During his day-long workshop on healing lower back pain with yoga, I was amazed by his depth of knowledge and overall presence. In his teacher training manual, he describes the system of yoga he created in this way:

> Purna means "complete" and Purna Yoga™ distills and integrates the vastness of yoga into an invaluable set of tools for transformation and healing. The lineage of Purna Yoga is based on the teachings of Sri Aurobindo and The Mother, the Vedas, Patanjali, B.K.S. Iyengar, and the systems of Ayurvedic, Chinese and Western nutrition, synthesized by the personal experience of Aadil Palkhivala and Savitri. It is the art of loving yourself and living from the heart. (Palkhivala 2008b, p.14)

I grabbed an application for his next 2000-hour teacher training program in Bellevue, Washington, uncertain of how I would manage to travel there four times every year. But somehow, despite the obstacles, I graduated from the College of Purna Yoga in 2006.

During my two decades of working with clients suffering physical injuries and chronic pain, I have noticed a common thread. Most of us have a feeling that "we are not good enough" and spend our lives trying to prove to ourselves that we are wrong. We approach life with a need to control it, and the need to be better than everyone else, while underneath it all, we also have a gnawing feeling that something is missing, or wrong. We may lack the awareness or sensitivity to hear what our hearts are trying to tell us, but nonetheless, there is a soft calling deep inside us that we cannot ignore, a voice telling us that there is another way to be in the world.

And that is why I have written this book—so that other yoga teachers, physical therapists, and medical and health professionals can better help their students and clients to heal themselves.

The lower back and sacrum make up the foundation of our spine. Our sense of survival is lodged there, as well as our root chakra, the energy center symbolizing our relationships, home, safety, money, and family. When we feel out of control in our lives, our spinal muscles contract to hold us together. In an attempt to survive, the sympathetic "fight or flight" nervous system fires continually, creating and maintaining tension throughout the body. In order to heal, it is important to allow ourselves to move from an anxious and high-tension mindset to a more expansive and trusting one.

What I have learned—after building up a lifetime of coping mechanisms to control my unstable surroundings—is that this type of living, of striving and gripping, of holding on tight, only creates more tension. Letting go and trusting is the hardest thing I have ever had to practice.

Yoga is a brilliant and beautiful science designed to create a strong, healthy spine. But the intention of the practice is to allow us the freedom to sit, be still, and get to know our real problem, the mind. Pain is an opportunity to stop, listen, and do something different. Pain is how our bodies scream out for us to pay attention, to stop forcing and to start feeling. So, while stretching our bodies in yoga, we are given the opportunity to discover our true selves, to take each breath as it comes and to be present in every moment.

Yoga has not only healed my back, it has healed my life. It has not only given me tools I can use to relieve pain and discomfort, it has given me tools to deal with the challenges of being human in an ever-changing world. Yoga builds inside of us a way to trust in the unfolding of life as it is and to see the beauty in each moment, even in our struggles and pain.

Most people tend to go to health professionals expecting them to provide the right "fix." What I have seen, as a physical therapist for the last two decades, is that *true healing is a partnership and a process. It requires commitment, practice, patience, and acceptance.*

Yoga offers much more than a set of postures or therapeutic exercises; it can show your students and clients a new way to live in the body. Instead of trying to mask pain or fight it, we learn to sit with it and let it unwind from the inside out. To do so takes both persistence and kindness. And a great deal of courage.

This book is an instructional manual to help you help your students and clients work through their injuries and heal their back pain, but it is also a memoir of healing. It is the story of the mind–body connection and how paying attention to your big toe mound can, in fact, change your life.

PART I

Principles and Practices of Yoga for a Happy Back

CHAPTER 1

Concepts in Yoga Therapy

**All illness is a function
of the loss of the inner smile.**
Aadil Palkhivala

Yoga differs from conventional therapeutic techniques in that it is a physical practice but also a path towards self-awareness and healing. Yoga philosophy can serve as a guide to your students and clients who face difficult life situations, including pain and suffering. The only requirement is their willingness to change and their commitment to practice. Once you ask your clients to embark on this journey, once their eyes have been opened, it will be hard for them to turn back towards a life of blissful ignorance, even if it may be more comfortable to remain in the dark.

More and more, yoga is being recognized as an effective method towards healing from chronic pain. Doctors are referring their patients to therapeutic yoga classes, and hospitals are offering yoga as part of their wellness programs, since it is a way to empower individuals to participate in their own healing process. This chapter introduces *seven basic principles* that I have found essential for true and complete healing to occur for your students and clients with back pain:

1. Change the story about the pain

2. Peel the onion

3. Find the balance between stability and mobility

4. Maintain the natural curves of the spine

5. Don't be afraid to move

6. Find the middle way

7. Learn how to heal.

20

1. Change the story about the pain

I manufacture tension.

Dan S.

Dan walked into my yoga class one morning and introduced himself. "I've only done yoga a few times before and I have had lower back, shoulder, and neck problems for the last 20 years. Do you think this class is appropriate for me?"

"You are in the right place," I reassured him. "This class is perfect for beginners and we can work with your injuries."

Dan was skeptical. He had been chief of a fire department for 30 years and was very used to being in control and fixing everyone else's problems. After retiring, he realized it was time to take care of himself for once; his body was complaining to him. He was experiencing tingling and numbness in both hands, with pain and muscle spasms in his right arm, shoulder, and neck. An MRI report revealed three herniated discs in his neck and one in the lower back. He had pain extending down the right leg to the foot, and slight weakness in his right lower extremity as well. An orthopedic surgeon had told him that "his life was over" and that he would most likely "end up being a quadriplegic. You'll be lucky if we can help you with surgery."

Dan decided to try other methods instead. While ordinary medicine could not heal him, he looked towards eastern philosophy for help. He began to come to my Happy Back yoga class every week. Shortly afterwards, he decided to come in for some private therapy. We slowly and methodically worked on opening up his chest, upper back, shoulders, hips, and neck with a combination of yoga practices and manual therapy. Dan reported that his muscle spasms stopped within the first month or two after beginning a regular yoga practice. He still complained of mild aches and pains, including neck tightness and shoulder impingement, but has not taken a pain pill or muscle relaxant since his first class.

Dan also began to get his "life" back. He returned to physical activity and began hiking five miles two to three times a week, swimming, and stand-up paddle boarding.

While this was going on, Dan began to notice changes that went way beyond those to his physical body. He became calmer and felt less need to control others. Just as I had learned to do, he began to slow down and take walks by the ocean every morning. He attended a conference on mindfulness. Slowly, he began to see what he felt was his purpose in this life. Dan decided that he wanted to help individuals in public safety recognize the benefits of a yoga practice in prolonging their careers, decreasing job-related injuries and improving their quality of life. He joined a course on Contemplative Dialogue with the intention of facilitating a dialogue between government agencies and the communities they serve. His relationship with his wife deepened as well when they began to practice deeper listening and acceptance, something Dan credits to his yoga and meditation practice and "taking a long, loving look at the real."

Dan is not alone. An increasing number of individuals have experienced profound shifts in their physical and emotional well-being, using the tools yoga has to offer as a path towards self-awareness and transformation. And for most, the motivation is pain.

Like Dan and me, several other clients discovered that pain could lead to positive changes in their lives.

- Lydia had shoulder and neck pain followed by debilitating migraines and eventually came to realize that her high-pressure job and perfectionist approach to life were literally killing her. After having to go on disability, she began to study yoga and practice Ayurveda; she left a destructive relationship and moved to a new city to find out what it really was that she wanted to do.

- Jack had back surgery for a herniated disc and came to physical therapy for residual back pain and numbness. Years later, he became a yoga instructor and moved away from his corporate construction job to focus on his dharma (life purpose): building sustainable projects in the US and India.

- Simon suffered from chronic pain and multiple injuries following a motorcycle accident at the age of 18; these prevented him from doing most physical activities he loved. He began a very limited and modified yoga practice along with physical therapy and found a new way to accept himself and be in his body. He went on to become a yoga instructor, and specializes in therapeutics as well. He works with children with special needs.

Pain can be a gateway

I have noticed that I am a more mindful and efficient swimmer when working against the current. For me, when the ocean is calm and peaceful, I tend to get a bit lazy, taking more breaks and stopping to look around and rest. When the current is against me, it gives me some resistance to work against. I therefore keep to a more steady rhythm, monitor my breath, and stay consistent with my strokes in order to forge ahead. For, if I don't work a little bit harder, the ocean will push me off course.

That has been true in my life as well. When things are going smoothly, I tend to enjoy it and am rarely motivated to focus on personal practice and spiritual growth. It has only been through pain and adversity that I have had to literally pick myself off the ground and take a huge step forward, followed by another and another, even though my legs felt like lead. I came to yoga in the wake of my first divorce, when I had not only let go of my husband, but of what seemed to be my entire belief system, religion, and social support network at that time. In choosing to forge my own path, I found myself out at sea with no buoy in sight, and was looking for something other than religion and marriage to help me find a sense of self that was then only a tiny flicker of possibility.

From my many personal experiences and from working with clients suffering from chronic pain and injuries, I have come to believe that injuries happen for a reason. Although it may not be apparent at the time, if you can step back and *reframe your pain* as an opportunity to look deeper, you can work on it with more acceptance, patience, and clarity. When your body sends a clear message, you are being given an invitation to re-examine the way you have been living your life physically, emotionally, and spiritually. This can point you in the direction of making changes, enabling you to achieve new levels of health and awareness.

My back injury certainly guided me to cease pushing toward my concept of perfection. It helped me learn to accept myself in this moment. It brought me face to face with my ego and insecurities. Though neither easy nor pleasant, I am grateful that my injury steered me towards a more compassionate way of living my life and practicing yoga.

It has also been my experience that the more I tried to mask the pain and deny it, the more it resurfaced with a vengeance. I always tell my clients that if they are experiencing an injury, they should consider themselves lucky. While this sounds strange, it is also true that pain can be a messenger telling them to stop and pay attention. They have the ability to improve their health and their lives if they listen and avoid more serious consequences.

Similarly, if your clients can change their view of pain, it can become a gift instead of a curse. This will help them feel more joy and compassion towards themselves and generate more patience for true healing.

There is a concept in yoga called Pratipaksha Bhavana, or the cultivation of opposite and uplifting emotions. This tool can help your clients reprogram their minds to replace negative thoughts with more positive emotions so that they can break free from habitual patterns of self-sabotage and destruction.

By employing it during the healing process, clients can transform anger, fear, and feeling like a victim to gratitude, acceptance, and compassion. It is hard, when anyone is in pain, to see the good that might come from the situation, but practicing Pratipaksha Bhavana can help your clients (and you!) surrender to the bigger picture with more calm and ease. When people are less tense, the nervous system moves into a more restful state, one in which the body can begin to heal itself.

On especially difficult days, I often swim out to the buoy and repeat this prayer that has saved me from much additional suffering:

> **God, grant me the serenity to accept
>   the things I cannot change,**
> **The courage to change the things I can**
> **And the wisdom to know the difference.**
> **Thy will, not mine, be done.**
>
> Alcoholics Anonymous

This helps me let go of the need to control my current situation and allows me to surrender a little bit more to the magic of the present moment.

My yoga teacher, Aadil Palkhivala, tells a story of his visit to a chiropractor after an acute bout of lower back pain. The pain was severe and Aadil went to the health practitioner to help him realign his spine. The chiropractor asked him many questions, all of which he answered in a pleasant tone with a gentle smile. Towards the end of the visit the doctor looked puzzled and spoke. "May I ask you a question?"

"Certainly," replied my teacher.

"A lot of people visit my office who are experiencing a great deal of pain. I wonder how you can still smile when all this is going on?"

Aadil smiled again and answered softly, "I have no choice about the pain, but I do have the choice to be happy." You, too, can convey this message to your clients.

PRACTICE TIP 1

Encourage your clients to change the story about their pain simply by changing the question. Instead of asking "Why is this happening to me?" have them ask themselves: "What can I learn from this?"

---

2. Peel the onion

Anna was an avid yoga practitioner and taught several classes a week when we met in an advanced teacher training. She was complaining of pain in her lower back after practicing and teaching her classes. We began to work on her practice in private sessions, pose by pose, and initially found a hamstring tendonitis and muscle spasm in her quadratus lumborum (QL), a muscle that attaches from the lower ribs to the pelvis. We worked on teaching her how to practice so that she did not overstrain her muscles and how to modify various poses that were causing her harm. We worked on stretches to relax the QL, and taught her how to engage her core properly so her back muscles weren't overcompensating for weak abdominals.

She began to improve gradually, but started to feel aches and pains in different areas. One week her hip would hurt on the left, and the next week her right side would be painful. We continued to investigate further. What we learned over the next year of working together was that there were many layers of dysfunction contributing to Anna's changing symptoms.

The body is a marvelous thing. If something is out of order, it will find a way to use a different part of the body to compensate and facilitate the action required at the time. The problem is that these compensatory mechanisms end up creating pain and injury, since they are not doing the job they were originally designed for.

For example: Imagine you are a coach and have two athletes, a long-distance runner and a sprinter. Your long-distance runner is out with the flu, so you send your sprinter on a 21-mile run as a substitute. He may be able to handle it for a little while, but after the fifth mile or so, he begins to cramp, slow down, and run out of breath. He was not trained for that kind of work and therefore will eventually burn out. His muscles have been developed for short, powerful sprints and have more fast-twitch (Type II) fibers than the slow-twitch (Type I) fibers, which are required for greater endurance and long-distance running.

The following attitude assessment may help your clients when they become frustrated by their limitations or, like Anna, by the slow pace of their healing.

PRACTICE TIP 2

ATTITUDE ASSESSMENT

Do you sense that you are becoming frustrated because you have not yet found a single technique, a kind of magic bullet or perfect pill that will heal you immediately? If so, remind yourself that healing is a process. You may uncover new areas of dysfunction or even have setbacks on your journey, but you can release fear and know that you are in control. Then recommit to developing the patience and perseverance that will carry you through toward true healing.

In Anna's case, we found a very unstable sacroiliac joint that kept shifting into different positions of dysfunction as she practiced a flow style of yoga which requires a great deal of movement into spinal flexion and extension. We modified her practice to one that focused on stability and strength with longer holds and fewer continuous motions (such as sun salutations). But then we had to go deeper and *correct her patterns of dysfunction*, slowly turning off the muscles that were overworking and straining and training new ones that were able to keep her pelvis aligned and stable.

In addition, during her time in physical therapy, she was forced to look at some challenges in her life as well. She began to realize that she felt unstable in her marriage as well as in her career path. She was also unhappy where she lived and missed the mountains and trees where she had grown up.

Her course of treatment was lengthy, but she remained committed, despite the frustration and grief over the loss of doing what she loved most. In time, with hard work, patience, and perseverance, she found a new way to be in her body that kept her pain at bay. She began to surf and snowboard again and now enjoys a different but meaningful yoga practice. She also divorced and moved to a new town, and works on helping others achieve optimum health with Ayurveda and yoga.

Anna's story is an example of how we can help clients keep peeling off layers in the body in order to discover the true source of pain and dysfunction. Once we guide a client to correct or realign one area, another pain may come up because we are uncovering the source of the problem. Our bodies compensate so much that the pattern of compensation may be what is initially causing the pain. Once the body begins to come back into alignment, deeper sources of pain may become apparent. With kindness, you can guide your students or clients to be patient and let those sources of pain come up. When the root of the problem presents itself, true healing can begin. Share the practice tip below with your students or clients.

PRACTICE TIP 3

If you are ready to heal, ask yourself if you are also ready to begin "peeling the layers of the onion." Are you really open to seeing where the source of your discomfort lies? Are you open to taking the first step, knowing that you may uncover some other areas of tightness and/or dysfunction? Are you committed to yourself and the journey of unfolding?

3. Find the balance between stability and mobility

We are born with a predisposition towards having tighter muscles and ligaments or looser ones. A woman may come to her first yoga class and bring her head to her knees in a forward bend, while another practitioner who has been a diligent yoga student for ten years may never get there. Genetics will often determine our limitations, whether we like it or not. In his 2009 study "Knee laxity tied to menstrual cycle," Kleinman concluded that women tend to be more flexible than men, due to increased levels of the hormone relaxin and other hormonal fluctuations during their menstrual cycle, as well as during pregnancy.

In a study published by the *Journal of Strength and Conditioning Research* (Hoge *et al.* 2010), it was found that men have a significantly higher incidence of musculoskeletal stiffness than women. Similarly Scerpelli, Stayer and Makhuli (2005) found that after performing a stretching protocol, women in their study had improved flexibility while the men did not. In their article in *Orthopedics*, they attributed this to the fact that women are more ligament dominant, while men are considered more muscle dominant.

People come to yoga thinking that if they cannot touch their toes, they are not good at it. In fact, it is actually much safer to be stiff than overly flexible. Having hypermobile joints puts that individual at more risk for damage and injury resulting from overstretching and hyperextension. Joints that tend to get injured from yoga due to hypermobility include the shoulders, the knees, the lower back, and the sacroiliac joint. The reason for this is that it is much easier to release into a pose than to have to resist moving to your limit, pull back, and then stabilize.

Ligament injuries are among the most common conditions encountered in private practice and are the primary cause of musculoskeletal pain. When a ligament is overstretched or experiences micro-tears, as researchers Hauser *et al.* reported in *The Open Rehabilitation Journal* (2013), abnormal force is transmitted through the joint, which, in turn, leads to joint damage, including osteoarthritis.

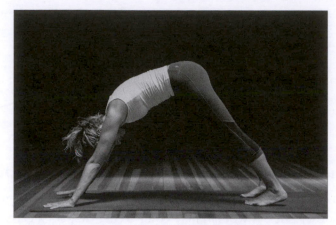

Figure 1.1 Adho Mukha Svanasana (AMS)/downward-facing dog (DD) with limited shoulder flexion

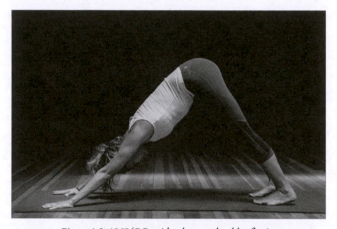

Figure 1.2 AMS/DD with adequate shoulder flexion

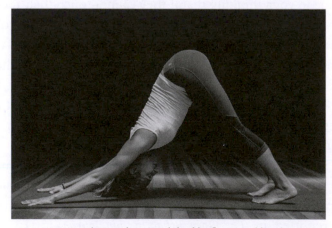

Figure 1.3 AMS/DD with increased shoulder flexion and hyperextension

My back injury and subsequent self-inquiry forced me to look closely and honestly at the way I was practicing yoga. I became aware that I was performing asana (postures) the way I thought they *should* look. I was missing an inner awareness of how each pose could serve my body and me. I would repeatedly overextend my lumbar spine while avoiding opening up tight areas in my body, namely my hip flexors and external hip rotators. My scoliosis also creates some restriction in my thoracic spine. In back bends, I continuously used the flexibility in my lower back to push into what I perceived was a deeper pose, instead of backing off to create more movement in my chest and upper back. In addition, I was not engaging my lower abdomen correctly, which contributed to constant compression in the lumbar spine. I was able to practice, even with this imbalance, for a number of years until the last straw broke the camel's back.

This is usually how an injury will occur; the muscles and joints slowly wear down until eventually something gives way.

The need for students and clients to achieve stability can be illustrated in downward-facing dog pose.

If the shoulders are above the torso (as in Figure 1.1), the individual needs to work on poses to open up the shoulders. Practicing Gomukhasana arms, the top arm specifically (see Figure 1.4), or half forward bend (see Figure 1.5) with hands on the wall, can have this opening effect. The individual can work on releasing into the pose to increase shoulder flexion.

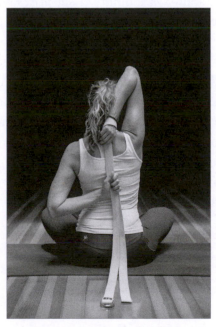

Figure 1.4 Gomukhasana/cowface pose

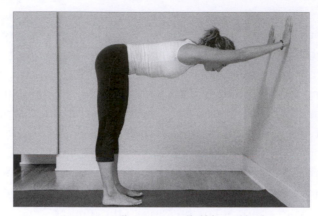

Figure 1.5 Ardha Uttanasana/half forward bend

If, however, the shoulder joint falls below the torso line, then the tendency for the student is to hyperextend at the shoulders, so she is essentially "sitting" on her shoulder joints (see Figure 1.3). Continuing to practice in this fashion will create repetitive shearing of the shoulder joint and will likely create impingement of the tendons (supraspinatus and long head of the biceps) in the joint. If the student has a tendency towards hypermobility, it is important for her to pull back from going to her end range of motion, and to stabilize the shoulder by focusing on moving the shoulder blade and the shoulder as one unit and activating the serratus anterior to spread the shoulder blades wide on the back.

Another common "stability vs. mobility" issue arises with the knee joint in standing poses. If the practitioner has average hamstring flexibility and good alignment in the knee joint, he can work on activating the quadriceps by lifting the kneecaps up into the thighs. Students who tend to hyperextend at the knee can damage the joint, since the tendency would be to "rest" on the ligaments instead of using the quadriceps muscle. For these individuals, it is essential that they micro bend the knee just enough so the joint is in neutral, and then work on contracting the quadriceps in this modified position (see Figure 1.6). Those of us who practice this way are well aware of how challenging it is to constantly maintain a balance between micro bending the knee and using the quadriceps at the same time.

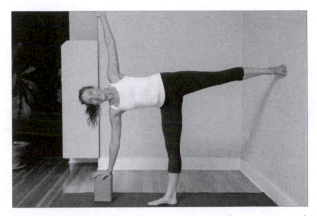

Figure 1.6 Ardha Chandrasana with knee micro bent while contracting quadriceps

One final example of the stability–mobility balance is the sacroiliac (SI) joint, which will be explored in more detail in Chapter 5.

When the SI joint is stable and there is little movement, there is little risk of injury. Pain and dysfunction in the SI joint occur when there is too much mobility, or an imbalance of mobility in the right vs. the left side. In yoga, those students with hypermobility will tend to have experiences in which the sacrum will go "out of joint" due to the constant movement of flexion to extension during sun salutations. The SI joint is also vulnerable during twists, for if there is limited rotation in the spine, especially the lumbar spine, the SI joint will rotate to compensate. This creates a shearing force in the joint, usually coupled with pain and decreased mobility. If the SI joint is out of place, it needs to be realigned; otherwise it will hurt in all poses. With the help of a skilled physical therapist, muscle energy techniques are extremely effective in realigning the sacrum, especially when followed by stabilization exercises.

Both the hip and shoulder joints are ball and socket joints, but differ considerably in their equation of stability vs. mobility due to their unique biomechanics (see Figure 1.7). The shoulder joint is designed for mobility. In order to provide increased mobility, the stability of the joint is sacrificed. This works well, since we don't usually stand and walk on our hands for most of the day. Conversely, our hips need to provide a great degree of stability for constant weight bearing and are therefore designed for less mobility; they are stabilized by a deep socket and multiple strong ligaments and muscles that surround the joint.

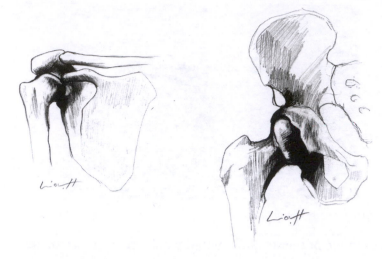

Figure 1.7 Increased stability in the hip joint vs. decreased stability in the shoulder joint

Given the difference between the hip and shoulder joints, it makes perfect sense that in guiding your students' yoga practice, you need to emphasize increasing *stability* in the shoulder and increasing *mobility* in the hip. As we learn in Purna Yoga, you should never stretch ligaments in your yoga practice, as they are designed to maintain the integrity of the skeleton. Overstretching can lead to instability and subsequent injuries.

One other important concept involving stability vs. mobility is individual difference. It is possible that for two different individuals the same yoga pose will need to focus on completely different instructions. So instead of trying to fit all your students or clients into a version of what you think the pose "should" look like, it is important to know the foundations of the pose, the intention, and the desired result, and then help the student or client find his or her natural alignment. Only then can you adapt the posture for their greatest benefit. This especially is why it is so important to have a solid foundation in alignment for any style of yoga practice.

Yoga is about balance. Always. And in this case we need to walk the fine line between increasing mobility and flexibility without losing integrity. This is the dance of yoga. Yin and Yang. The balance of containment and expansion, feminine and masculine, receiving and giving. It is the dance of life. Here is a practice tip that will help your students become more self-aware.

PRACTICE TIP 4

Decide which category you fall into. Be honest with yourself. Do you have loose ligaments and tend towards hyperextension in your joints, or do you feel somewhat restricted by tightness in your ligaments and muscles?

If you tend to be more flexible, focus on strength and stability in each pose. If you tend to be tighter, focus on lengthening and releasing into your postures.

Example: Supported lunge

- *To increase flexibility:* While keeping the knee directly above the ankle for safety, sink into the pose, emphasizing the releasing, softening, and opening of the hip flexors in the back leg (see Figure 1.8).

- *To increase stability:* Avoid going into your end range in the pose. Press the front foot and back shin into the ground. Back off a little and squeeze the inner thighs towards each other (see Figure 1.9).

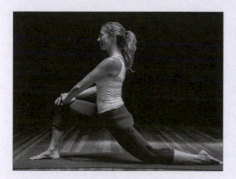

Figure 1.8 Supported lunge with emphasis on flexibility

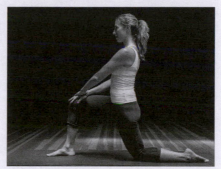

Figure 1.9 Supported lunge with emphasis on stability

4. Maintain the normal curves in the spine

**If you go against your nature, you suffer.
Find your natural grace.**

Judith Hanson Lasater (2005)

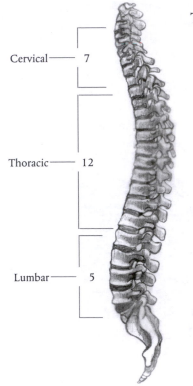

Cervical ——— 7

Thoracic ——— 12

Lumbar ——— 5

*Figure 1.10 Natural
spinal curves*

The spine is designed to absorb the weight of the world, which is not an easy task. Gravity is continually acting on us as we move about our daily tasks and activities. The primary way that the spine can rise to the challenge for so many years is by means of its structural curves. The primary curve is a kyphosis, as we are flexed in the uterus as infants. As we begin to exercise head control, our cervical spine develops a lordotic curve, followed by the lumbar lordosis when we begin crawling and walking. The curves are illustrated in Figure 1.10.

The natural curves of the spine help to absorb some of the load and distribute it throughout the spinal column. Any deviation from this ideal alignment will have an impact on how and where weight is transmitted through your student's vertebrae. If a spine is too straight, it creates too much stress on the already fragile lower spine and pelvis.

Consider the examples below.

a. Forward head posture

This posture is common in anyone who works for multiple hours sitting at a desk or computer. The head juts forward, causing the shoulders to round and the front of the chest to tighten. The lower cervical spine is in flexion while the upper cervical spine is in extension, in order to be able to lift the head up to see straight ahead. The upper back is weak and the postural muscles around the scapulae are stretched out. These changes eventually lead to chronic upper back and neck tension due to the muscles working harder to hold the head and back up. Other complications from adopting this posture include nerve impingement in the cervical

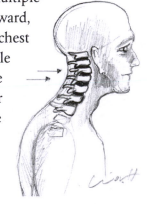

*Figure 1.11
Forward head posture*

spine due to less space in between the vertebrae; thoracic outlet syndrome from tightness in the chest; and carpal tunnel syndrome, as the blood flow and nerve conduction are impaired due to tightness in the anterior chest musculature and underarm area.

b. Decreased lumbar curve

This posture is common in men who also spend a lot of time sitting down. The decreased lumbar curve is largely due to tightness in the hamstrings, which pull the pelvis into a posterior tilt (Figures 1.12 and 1.13). This causes the normal lordosis of the lumbar spine to be reduced and creates a sense of "sitting on the lower back," tucking of the tailbone, loss of height in the spine, and a weak core. Further postural accommodations can include tightness in the hip external rotators and weakness in the inner thighs and pelvic floor, which is a recipe for compression in the lower back and sacroiliac joint. Common complications from this posture include disc bulge and herniation, as well as sciatica.

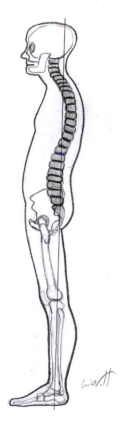

Figure 1.12
Decreased lumbar curve

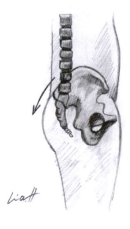

Figure 1.13 Posterior pelvic tilt

c. Decreased thoracic and cervical curve

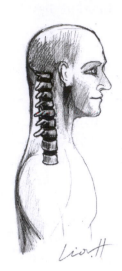

This posture is common in yoga practitioners. Sometimes, in the effort to open the chest, we forget to maintain the normal curves of the neck and back, and the spine becomes "too straight," or loses its curves. This creates a great deal of chronic pain, with tension in the upper back and neck, and can only be ameliorated by poses that soften the thoracic spine and maintain a natural lordotic curve in the neck.

Figure 1.14 Decreased thoracic and cervical curve

These following kinds of poses can help normalize spinal curves:

1. *Tadasana:* Tadasana, also known as mountain pose, is the foundational pose from which all other poses are modeled. It is where we learn how to correctly activate the feet and legs in both standing poses and inversions. We learn to lift the lower belly in order to support the spine and begin to activate the integrity of the core. We also learn how to let the shoulder blades drop away from the ears, in order to create less tension in the neck and more openness in the chest. In Tadasana we learn how to maintain the natural curvature of the spine (Figure 1.15).

2. *Forward bends:* In forward bends it is important to instruct students to maintain the lumbar curve by keeping the sacrum in line with the lumbar spine. This requires the practitioner to maintain an anterior pelvic tilt (Figure 1.16) while forward bending, an action that is commonly limited by tightness in the hamstrings.

3. *Back bends:* In back bends, there are two important things for your students or clients to keep in mind (Figure 1.17):

   a. Guide them to think about creating *length* along with extension in the spine. The most common error in these poses is that individuals tend to hinge at the lower back at one level. You might use the image of a string of pearls, encouraging students or clients to imagine each vertebra extending to form a beautiful and even arc. One way to accomplish this is to focus on maintaining length in the front body as you arch the back body.

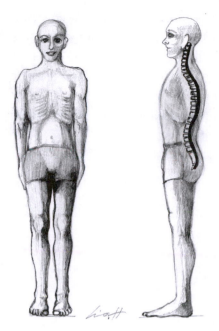

Figure 1.15 Tadasana/mountain
pose with natural spinal curves

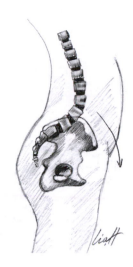

Figure 1.16 Anterior pelvic tilt

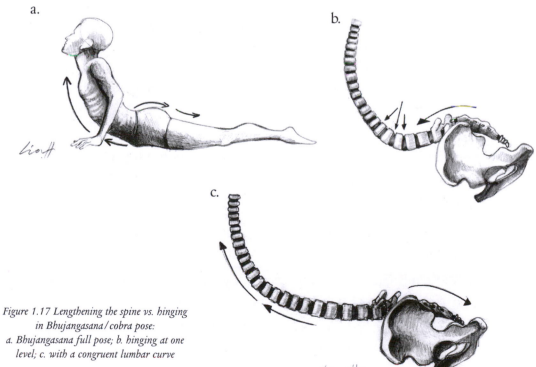

a.

b.

c.

Figure 1.17 Lengthening the spine vs. hinging
in Bhujangasana/cobra pose:
a. Bhujangasana full pose; b. hinging at one
level; c. with a congruent lumbar curve

b. When your students are doing a back bend, *they should do a back bend!* Extension is a normal range of motion for the spine and it is important, and safer, if you commit to that action. In order to encourage more spinal extension, ask them to feel as if their vertebrae are moving into their body, level by level with each exhalation. (See Chapter 1, Figure 1.18 and Chapter 3, Figures 3.6 and 3.7.)

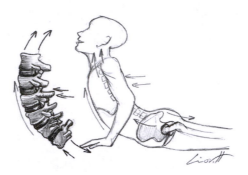

Figure 1.18 Bringing the spinous processes into the body in back bends

4. *Twists:* Twists naturally create a decrease in height of the spine due to the inherent body mechanics that occur during spinal rotation. In order to help students avoid compression, which can happen as we twist, guide them always to lengthen first on the inhalation, keeping the chest open, and then twist on the exhalation, while engaging the navel towards the lower back in order to activate the deeper abdominal muscles.

The basic take-home message is: Your students should understand the normal range of motion in their spine and know and commit to proper alignment in order to accomplish each movement safely. You can help them to:

- know when they are doing a back bend or forward bend

- avoid turning standing poses into back bends. Instead, maintain core awareness with an emphasis on lifting the lower belly

- understand that more is not necessarily better—ask them to maintain *integrity* in the pose

- avoid hinging at one level (which will be their weakest link). Try to open the tight areas. Practice with more awareness.

You can ask your students and clients to practice proper standing with the following tip.

PRACTICE TIP 5

Stand in Tadasana (mountain pose)—have a partner apply gentle pressure to your shoulders in a downward direction. Notice if you collapse forward or backwards, or if you feel steady. Then make some adjustments:

- draw the shoulder blades away from the ears
- roll the thighs inward, relaxing the buttocks
- lift the lower belly towards your chin
- make sure there is equal weight in all four corners of the feet.

Now retest. We are looking to find the place where you feel completely stable while maintaining the natural curves of the spine. Practice regularly to create muscle memory and integrate this awareness into your nervous system.

You can teach your students and clients to practice proper standing by using The Vertebral Compression Test on page 64.

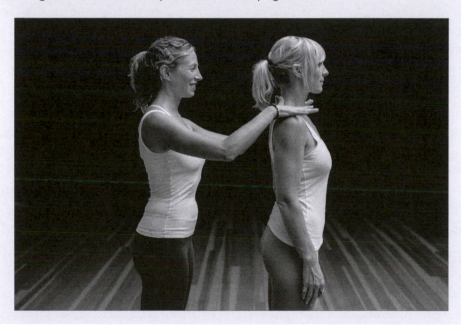

5. Don't be afraid to move

When I herniated my disc, my doctor told me I would have to "modify my activities for the rest of my life." I feel lucky that I knew better instinctively, but many of my patients have had fear instilled in them that they will break if they move. You will give your students and clients valuable practical wisdom when you tell them: *"Know that things go terribly wrong when we stop moving."* The body is inherently designed to nourish itself with synovial fluid, which gets pushed around in the joints when we move. When we stay still, the joints dry out, muscles atrophy and tighten up around the joints, and the tissue degenerates. The old saying "Use it or lose it" should be the motto for the body. The body adapts to the forces that are applied to it. Our bones get stronger only with weight applied to them, muscles stay supple and long when they are continually stretched, and joint mobility is largely dependent on moving the joint.

I recently tore a tendon in my middle finger and had to wear a splint for six weeks in order for the connective tissue to regenerate. After I removed the splint, I was surprised at how stiff the tiny joint in my finger had become. Everything had tightened up and it was a painful process to get it to start working again, which required directed effort and exercise. While this was a minor injury, it reminded me how thankful we should be for all the parts that move without effort. An entire system is at work to keep us mobile and functional; we often take that system for granted.

For instance, a part of this system is a very small structure in the facet joints (the joints of the spine) called the *meniscoid structure*. In addition to filling in the incongruence in the joint surfaces, Czech researchers Kos, Hert and Sevcík (2002) explained in their "Meniscoids of the intervertebral joints" that these structures are responsible for the transportation of synovial fluid around the joints occurring with movement. The meniscoids act like a "squeegee system" to keep the joint juicy and to prevent degeneration. Think of the synovial fluid as WD-40 for your students' and clients' joints. Your own, too!

The mechanism for disc injuries is usually in the area of the disc which did not get enough hydration and therefore dried up and cracked, allowing the nucleus pulposus (the jelly-like disc material in the center) to seep into the cracks of the annulus fibrosus and eventually make its way out. That is why physical therapists will evaluate joint mobility at each level of the spine to find out which segments are not moving correctly. The treatment is to correct any movement dysfunctions so that there is balanced movement in all directions and each joint can be nourished.

Of course, that doesn't mean that you should advise your students to go out and run a marathon after being diagnosed with degenerative disc disease. Rest is important during the acute phases of any inflammatory condition. However, smart, mindful, and appropriate movement will heal your clients over the long term. The challenge comes in knowing what to tell them to do at what stage in their healing process. They are already working with you, a trained professional, which is the best way to get started. You can help them to realize that they will not be limited forever. Keep reminding them that they will move again, and have them picture themselves doing the activities they love. They may need to change or alter some of those activities, but they can always live a vibrant, active life. And encourage them to know that they may learn something new in the process.

When I herniated my disc, I wondered if I would ever get to practice yoga again. Now, a decade later, I enjoy a full practice but still have to be very conscious about the sequencing and instructions I follow. Another opportunity for self-awareness…sigh.

6. Find the middle way

> **Your hand opens and closes and opens and closes.**
> **If it were always a fist or always stretched**
> **open, you would be paralyzed.**
> **Your deepest presence is in every small**
> **contracting and expanding,**
> **The two as beautifully balanced**
> **and coordinated as birdwings.**
>
> Rumi

Yoga is about finding a balance. Similarly, the body wants to attain balance—physically and physiologically—at all times. One of the best and most striking examples of this is found in individuals with scoliosis. If a primary curve is side bent to the right and rotated to the left, the vertebrae above and below the curve will adapt to compensate for this unusual alignment and side bend, and rotate in the opposite direction. The spine will do whatever it needs to do to literally keep your head on straight. I even noticed that my jaw and facial bones had adjusted to compensate for the scoliosis I had in my thoracic spine!

Knowing that the body is seeking balance and alignment naturally helps us approach teaching students and treating clients in a different way. With this concept in mind, healing becomes less about changing your students' or clients' bodies and more about *releasing the blockages* so that each of their spines can find its own balance and lengthen. Just as the sculpture is already in the stone, waiting for the sculptor to take away the unnecessary stone, to reveal the inherent beauty, we can remove the excess tension that is pulling the spine out of alignment. Then the spine will be free to lengthen and find its natural curve. This is a common concept in yoga, which is ultimately a way of cleaning out the "junk" in our minds and bodies in order to reveal the true Self.

Blockages can include lack of motion or a joint being "stuck" so that it is not following the rhythm of the body. It can also include tight muscles and connective tissue that can create compression in the joints they traverse. Once again, fostering self-awareness will help your students know which muscles to stretch and which to strengthen, as well as which joints to mobilize and which to stabilize. Once each of your clients knows his or her self and body in this intimate way, a feeling of empowerment follows and healing is just around the corner.

7. Learn how to heal

With back pain, individuals usually skip steps when working on the healing process. There is a huge emphasis on strengthening the core, which is indeed very important for back health. However, strengthening a structure that is not properly aligned will not correct the problem. It is like building a fence around a house with a crooked foundation. It is essential that the source of the pain or dysfunction be exposed and corrected before effective stabilization can occur. Below are the stages of healing that are necessary for complete recovery.

The five stages of healing

1. *Realign:* Identify what is tight and what is weak and work on correcting both.

2. *Create space:* Open up the tight structures and surrounding connective tissue to reduce joint and nerve compression.

3. *Re-educate:* Identify faulty movement patterns that contribute to the imbalances and learn how to move in a different way.

4. *Stabilize:* Align the structure first, then stabilize.

5. *Practice:* Be consistent for long-term results and transformation. Guide your students to make their practice a good habit, like brushing their teeth.

Conclusion and case study

All these recommendations address injuries solely on the physical level. In order to fully heal, it is important to address all of the five *koshas*, or "sheaths," of the body. In yoga philosophy, the koshas relate to the physical body (*annamaya kosha*), the energy body (*pranamaya kosha*), the mental/ emotional body (*manomaya kosha*), the wisdom body (*vijnanamaya kosha*) and the bliss body (*anandamaya kosha*).

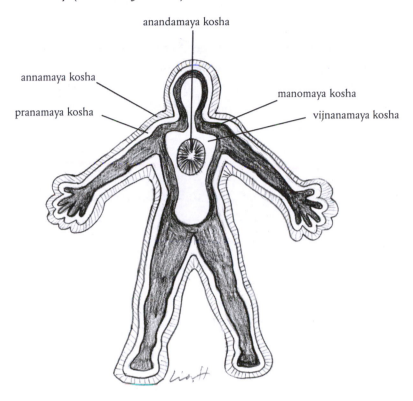

Figure 1.20 Diagram of the five koshas

To help heal others, we need not move in numerical order through all five levels, but rather, we guide them to work on all levels simultaneously to promote complete healing. Unfortunately, like most things that are worthwhile, this takes hard work, commitment, and patience. There is no magic pose or quick fix. Rather, each journey is as unique as each person's own individual landscape. There are many ways to get to the same place. Listed below are some active techniques to offer students and clients from your healing palette. Encourage them to do the following:

1. Pay attention! The body is asking that they stop and change something. Don't just power through the pain. Ask, "What can I learn from this?"

2. Move mindfully: Begin a physical practice that focuses on awareness and breath.

3. Meditate regularly to achieve mindfulness and presence.

4. Change their diet: Nutrition and lifestyle practices are crucial to the healing process. They may consult an Ayurvedic practitioner who will make recommendations suited to their unique constitution and lifestyle.

5. Explore their emotional landscape: Perhaps advise them to consult with a psychotherapist or counselor to uncover deeper causes of pain, both physical and emotional. Until this piece is really addressed, complete healing cannot happen. The body tends to reflect the inner tension of the mind. If students do not face these demons, they tend to get stronger.

6. Be kind to themselves: Move away from any self-judgment or criticism. See this process as an opportunity to be more patient with themselves. As Judith Hanson Lasater (2005) says, "May we be like the lotus, at home in the muddy water."

7. Address the nervous system: One of the main beneficial effects of regular yoga practice is on the nervous system. Yoga moves us from a stress response to a more calm and relaxed state in which the body can heal. There are many other complementary modalities that help us address our bodies on a cellular level as our bodies process tension that we cannot reach through the intellect. Examples of these modalities include yoga nidra (guided relaxation), somatic experiencing, acupuncture, restorative yoga, craniosacral therapy, Traumatic Releasing Exercises (TRE), and time in nature.

8. Look inward. There is no end point, as this is a process that continues through life. Students and clients must continue to pay attention to the messages they receive from their bodies and make continual adjustments. The more sensitive they become, the more readily they can respond to their own inner wisdom.

CASE STUDY: MARK

Background

Mark is a 45-year-old computer programmer who spends eight hours a day sitting in front of the computer. He has a flat lower back with tight hamstrings and hip flexors. His head sits forward and his shoulders are rounded, which leads to a weak upper back and tight chest muscles. His core is weak as he spends most of his day sitting at a desk and only occasionally runs on the weekends. He feels stuck at his job but does not know what he wants to do in the future. Well into his career, it is hard for him to imagine a change, yet he remains dissatisfied and stays in his job for security and the health/retirement package.

Mark bent down to pick up a piece of paper from the floor and felt a shooting pain down his right leg. Shortly afterwards, he was unable to stand up straight. He went to the doctor and received anti-inflammatory medication and was offered a steroid injection. An MRI scan revealed a disc bulge with nerve root impingement on the right. He was told to rest and return in six weeks for follow-up and possible pre-op evaluation.

Mark spent one week on the floor lying on his belly, which provided him with some temporary relief. He was unable to sit for longer than five minutes without back and leg pain, and he was experiencing pins and needles in his right foot.

We will be following Mark's journey toward healing and wholeness throughout the chapters of this book.

CHAPTER 2

Functional Anatomy

Structure, Movement, and Screening the Spine

**Our bodies tell the story
that we are trying to hide.**
Rachel Krentzman

Two factors distinguish yoga therapy from most orthopedic approaches to spinal health. The first is a strong emphasis on *function* and movement, rather than simply on anatomy and structure; the second is an emphasis on the Ayurvedic concept of the five koshas, also known as energetic layers or sheaths. Yoga therapy integrates its exploration of functional movement and the five koshas, especially the emotional and spiritual components, into evaluation and treatment planning; it takes a holistic and multifaceted approach to healing.

Before exploring yoga-based practices for back pain, you need to have a good understanding of anatomy and biomechanics, as well as a basic knowledge of common pathologies of the spine and pelvis. The essential transformation that occurs in a client's yoga practice goes far beyond the physical realm; but, when working with patients with back pain, you will need to know a great deal more about the body than most studio yoga instructors. The deeper your understanding of the physical body and how it moves, the more you will be able to safely help students and clients with back pain and common spinal conditions.

In this chapter we will also explore other concepts missing from many anatomy books; concepts that hold the key to understanding why so many individuals have pain despite their lack of obvious physical disabilities— and why others with significant dysfunction or anomalies on diagnostic imaging can live full, active lives without pain. John Sarno (1991), in his controversial and revolutionary book *Healing Back Pain*, argues against the generally accepted wisdom that relates changes on X-rays, CT scans, or MRI scans to the patient's level of pain. Sarno proceeds condition by condition, showing that each common spinal diagnosis is not a reliable indicator of a certain level of pain or disability. While his approach is difficult for many medical professionals to accept, many other studies support his finding that back pain is not necessarily proportional to the severity of physical anomalies found on imaging. Among these studies supportive of Dr. Sarno's work are: Deyo and Weinstein (2001) in *The New England Journal of Medicine*; Borenstein *et al.* (2001) in the *Journal of Bone and Joint Surgery*; Haig *et al.* (2006) in the *Archives of Physical Medicine and Rehabilitation*; Bogduk (2000) in *The Medical Journal of Australia*; and Jensen *et al.* (1994) in *The New England Journal of Medicine*.

Two principles explaining this disparity have helped me treat individuals with back pain. The first is the concept of *structural vs. movement dysfunction* that we will explore in depth in this chapter. The second involves the *emotional and spiritual factors* that contribute to pain; these factors will be addressed in greater detail in Chapter 8.

Anatomy of the spine

As noted in Chapter 1, the three main curves of the normal spine are the cervical lordosis, thoracic kyphosis, and lumbar lordosis. These are formed by seven cervical, twelve thoracic, and five lumbar vertebrae. The sacrum itself has five levels, which are fused into one bone that sits at a 30° angle to the horizontal line. The presence of this angle is important because the properly angled sacrum helps create the pelvic cavity and provides support to the abdominal and pelvic organs, as well as the lower back and pelvic floor musculature.

As babies in the womb, we have one primary spinal curve, a kyphosis that resembles the position of the spine in child's pose (Figure 2.2). Perhaps this is why this pose is so comforting to all of us. It reminds us of a time in our lives when we were safe and supported. It is also a posture that stimulates the parasympathetic, or relaxation, response.

As the baby begins to lift its head while in a prone position, the cervical curve begins to develop, and subsequently the lumbar curve develops when the child starts standing and walking. The important thing to remember is that these curves are normal and they exist to help absorb the load imposed on the spine by standing, sitting, and moving, and to decrease the pressure on the most vulnerable part of the body, the lower lumbar spine, the vertebrae named L4–L5 and L5–S1.

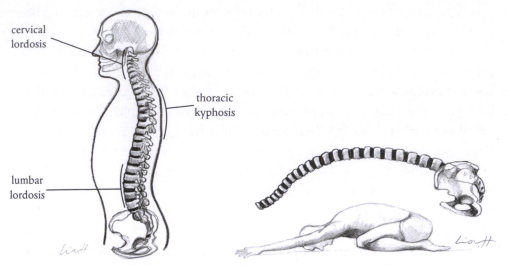

Figure 2.1 The spinal curves   Figure 2.2 Primary spinal curve (kyphosis)

Problems can arise when these curves are exaggerated, and also when the curves of the spine are lost and become too straight. We often think that a straighter spine is a healthier spine but, according to my clinical observations, this is not the case. In fact, I have worked with a great many yoga practitioners, teachers, and dancers who—over many years of these physical practices— have flattened out their curves in all areas of the spine. Such individuals usually have a good deal of pain and tension, especially in the upper back, neck, and shoulders, from the lack of softness and increased rigidity in the muscles, bones, and tissues. In further chapters, you will learn that some of these curves can be restored through yoga, if practiced mindfully and with clear intention to normalize the curves.

In Tadasana, the natural curves of the spine should be maintained *while lengthening and maintaining space between each pair of vertebrae.* Many individuals squeeze their buttocks in this pose and attempt to "tuck the tailbone" under. This action eliminates the healthy lumbar curve that helps to support the spine, organs, and pelvic floor. Instead it is better to "lift the lower belly" or, as my teacher Aadil Palkhivala calls it, "the pit of the abdomen" (POA). This action helps to eliminate any excessive curvature in the lower back, while creating length and space between each vertebra. It also takes the focus off the tailbone and brings more awareness to the front of the body and the often weak abdominals.

Still, it is not possible to maintain the natural curves of the spine in all postures, for in yoga we take the spine into many extremes of ranges of motion.

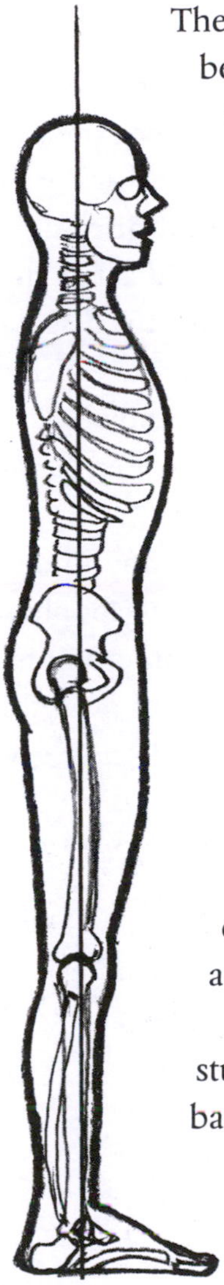

The basic concept is that if the spine is in a neutral position, it is best to try to maintain the natural curvature as much as possible so that gravitational forces are distributed throughout the body in a healthy way. You can measure this by using a yoga strap while assessing your clients' posture in standing and in Tadasana. Simply hold the strap in the area of the center of the ear and see where it falls. It should fall through the center of the ear, center of the shoulders and waist, center of the hip joint, just a little anterior to the knee joint, and anterior to the ankle joint and the lateral malleolus (heel) bone (see Figure 2.3).

Students or clients may think that their lumbar curves are too large and, therefore, may try to minimize them. In truth, most individuals do not have *enough* of a curve in their lower backs. To counteract this common misperception, I have found from evaluating many different bodies that two instructions are most crucial in mountain pose—to roll the skin of the inner thighs backwards (slight internal rotation at the level of the hips) and to lift the lower belly (the pit of the abdomen). These two actions, while difficult to accomplish at the same time, create more length in the lumbar spine while helping to maintain a natural lumbar curve.

A third instruction that I find important to impart to my students is to "deepen the groins" and take the tops of the thighs back. If done correctly, this action creates softness in the hip creases and will also help to facilitate the normal lumbar curve. When instructing your students, ask them to push their thighs forward and see the creases in the groin disappearing and hardening. Then have them do the opposite action and move the tops of the thighs back. Teach them to look at their pants so that they can see a crease emerging in the groin area; ask them to note the softness in the hip flexors. Pushing the hips forward makes the groins hard and increases tension in the iliopsoas muscles and the rectus femoris (one of the four quadriceps). Such tension in the hip flexors, especially the psoas major, has a direct effect on spinal health because the hip flexors attach to the lumbar vertebrae and discs, exerting a muscular pull and potentially causing compression, an anterior tilt, and back pain (see Figure 2.4 a.).

Figure 2.3 The plumb line—where gravity should fall in relation to the spine and extremities

Range of motion in the spine

Before discussing the actual movement that we can expect to see at the various levels of the spine, we need to understand where, in a healthy spine, the movement actually occurs. Most individuals think that the discs are the joints in the spine, but this is not the case. The intervertebral discs do not move—they join each vertebra to the ones above and below and act as shock absorbers for the spine. Movement in the spine helps to nourish the discs, and conversely, lack of movement causes the discs to dry up and crack, which can lead to disc bulges and herniations down the road. With this knowledge we can see that *the body is designed for movement* and that *health is directly proportional to activity*, especially as we age.

The actual movement at each vertebral level occurs at two tiny joints on each vertebral segment; these are called the "facet joints" or "zygapophyseal joints" (see Figure 2.4 b.). These joints, while small, are the only points on each vertebral segment where movement occurs. They consist of everything a larger joint has, including a joint capsule and synovial fluid, along with cartilage that lines the top of each joint surface.

a.

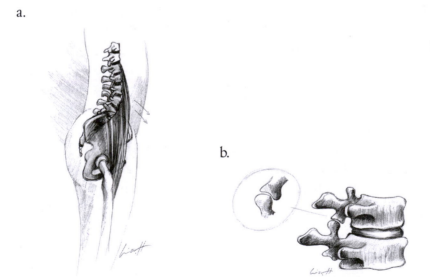

b.

Figure 2.4 a. The pull of the hip flexors on the lumbar spine; b. the facet joints of the lumbar spine

The shape and surfaces of the facet joints change as we move down the spine from the cervical to the lumbar region. These anatomical differences affect the range of motion at each spinal level. The facet joints are not ball and socket joints such as those in the hip and shoulder; in contrast, facet joints have a limited range of motion. Their movement consists of gliding either forward (into flexion) or backwards (into extension). The shape of these joints relative to the level above or below dictates how many degrees of movement are available in the spine at that level and what restrictions will be present during various yoga postures.

The cervical spine has the most mobility, as the facet joints rest one on top of the other at a relatively horizontal angle. Consequently, there is approximately 50° of flexion, 60° of extension, 45° of lateral bending, and 80–90° of rotation available in the neck. In the thoracic spine, there is about 50° of thoracic forward bending and lateral flexion as well as a fair amount of rotation available (approximately 30–45°). Thoracic extension (back bending) is quite limited by both the long spinous processes and the fact that the rib cage is attached to the vertebrae of the upper back, contributing to decreased mobility. This limitation is present for a very good reason. It creates protection for the most essential and most delicate organ, the heart. The rib cage and the thoracic spine protect the heart from harm. This protection is crucially present in a healthy upper body, but a tight chest and restricted rib cage and thoracic spine can come about as a means of "closing off" or "guarding" the heart excessively due to past hurt or trauma. This is often why working on back bends and chest opening can cause a great deal of emotion to come to the surface. Opening the chest is literally a means of opening your heart as well.

In the lumbar spine, there is 60–90° of flexion, 30° of extension, and 20–45° of lateral flexion. The movement that is most limited in the lumbar area is rotation; the angle of the facet joints of the spine restricts rotation to a maximum of 10–15° throughout the entire lumbar area.

Magnetic resonance imaging (MRI) has underscored these findings about the normal spine. Ryaturo (2007), in his "Kinematics of the lumbar spine in trunk rotation," found that the total degree of trunk rotation is approximately 45° in the thoracic region and approximately 10° in the lumbar region, which suggests that trunk rotation occurs predominantly in the thoracic region rather than in the lumbar region. This is largely due to the dramatic changes in the angle of the facet joints from more frontally oriented in the thoracic spine to more medially oriented in the lumbar spine.

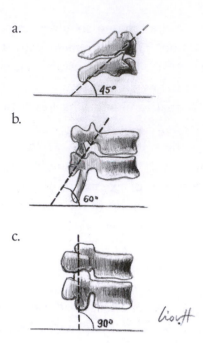

Figure 2.5 The angles of the facet joints in: a. cervical spine; b. thoracic spine; c. lumbar spine

It is important to understand the way the joints of the spine are designed and how they move; having this knowledge can positively affect your ability to teach and guide students through their asana practice. For example, if you understand that the lumbar spine is limited to 10–15° of rotation and that most of the rotation in the spine happens in the thoracic spine, you will make sure to avoid forcing more twist in the lumbar area and, instead, encourage rotation to come from the upper back. Forcing a twist or adjusting a student in an aggressive way by rotating their shoulders in a seated spinal twist can cause damage to the joints of the lumbar spine, as they may experience compression and subsequent inflammation and/or pain in this area. Yes, we do want to lengthen the lumbar spine before we twist, and it is appropriate to adjust the student's sacrum to lift and move it into the body to encourage the natural lumbar curve, but it is never correct to adjust students by twisting them from the outside in by holding onto their shoulders.

a. 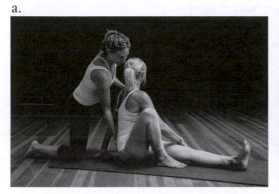 b.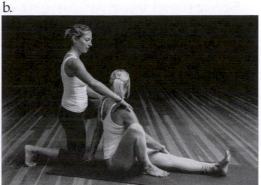

Figure 2.6 a. Proper adjustment during spinal twist using the hand on the student's sacrum;
b. incorrect adjustment in a twist

Similarly, when working with back bends, we need to understand the anatomy and biomechanics of the spine. Students are often concerned about hurting their backs in these poses. The reality is that forward bends are actually more risky than back bends. Why? *Because the lower back is designed to do back bends.* There is a great deal of extension in the lumbar spine, and it is considered a normal movement for the spine. Excessive forward bending, on the other hand, can put additional pressure on the discs and can be the cause of a disc herniation or bulge.

While the lower back can move readily into extension, the upper back tends to be more limited due to the anatomy of the thoracic vertebrae. When you know this, then you will encourage the student to open the upper back as much as possible while allowing the back bend to come from the lumbar area as well. Very often people are afraid of overextending the lumbar spine and, because of that, they fight going into extension in that area while in a back bend. As mentioned in Chapter 1, back bends are actually safe and good for the lower back (in most cases) and are best practiced by allowing the lumbar spine to move fully into extension. The key here, and the issue that has generally arisen when people get pain in their lower back, is that they are not maintaining length in the lower back while extending, but rather are *hinging at one level.* In essence, many individuals are actually doing a forward bend in their back bends. In a back bend, it is much safer and more natural to move the spine into the body and embrace the extension component of the lumbar spine, as illustrated in Chapter 3, Figures 3.6 and 3.7.

Structural vs. movement dysfunction

Now that we have seen the basic structure of the spine and its various ranges of motion, we can begin to understand one of the main reasons why there is often, as Dr. Sarno discovered, a wide discrepancy between pain and actual changes revealed by diagnostic imaging. Such images, whether by X-ray, CT, or MRI, are taken while the patient is in a static position. And so we see a picture of the spine in only one position, with no record of movement. Such images do not provide a functional measurement. Most individuals who come in for treatment find that their spines look normal on an X-ray or MRI, and yet they are experiencing a great deal of pain during certain movements.

In his *Lumbo-Pelvic Integration* manual (2006), physical therapist Jeffrey Ellis introduces the premise that "The musculo-skeletal system functions as one large kinetic chain with multi-segmental contributions." This reiterates an idea that is integral to yoga and yoga therapy; that *each part of the body is affected by and affects the rest of the body*. Yoga philosophy goes even further, understanding that the body is not only one kinetic chain in terms of its physical elements, but that every aspect of the individual's being—all five of the koshas—affects every other.

This brings us to the functional anatomy of yoga, a holistic approach that uses the kosha model as a means towards understanding the health and well-being of each individual. In yoga philosophy, the koshas are the five "sheaths" or layers of being, the innermost of which is the true Self called *anandamaya kosha*, meaning the bliss of union with the true Self and all that is. The other layers are: the mortal, physical body which is fed by food and is called *annamaya kosha*; the energy body fed by *prana* (our life force or vital principle) and called *pranamaya kosha*; the mind fed by the sense organs and called *manomaya kosha*; and finally, the intellect fed by perception and knowledge and called the *vijnanamaya kosha*. The aim of yoga and yoga therapy is to come back to the deepest layer, the core self that is *ananda* (bliss) inside each of us. We do this by healing, transcending, and/or balancing out any dysfunction or dissonance in the other koshas. When using this approach, we do not work in a linear model, moving from superficial to deep, but rather in a fully integrative and holistic way. We are always exploring and working on all five sheaths at the same time. Only if all aspects of a student or patient's being are addressed can that person heal fully from physical, mental, and emotional pain and find freedom from suffering despite outside circumstances.

When we approach pain from this model, we understand that we cannot address only our student or client's physical body. I have seen over and over again that if someone has pain in one area of the body and "fixes" the physical problem without addressing other aspects of his or her life, the pain will appear somewhere else. The body will keep sending messages in different forms until the individual "gets it" and takes a long, close look at what the true source of pain is in all aspects of his or her being. As B.K.S. Iyengar states in his *Light on Life* (2005):

> When these subtle sheaths are in disharmony, they become sullied like a mirror reflecting the tarnished images of the sensory and sensual world. The mirror reflects what is in the world around us rather than letting the clear light of the soul within shine out. It is then that we experience disease and despair. True health requires not only the effective functioning of the physical exterior of our being, but also the vitality, strength, and sensitivity of the subtle levels within. (Iyengar 2005, p.4)

Using the kosha model, when we evaluate the physical level (*annamaya kosha*), we can readily see that there is often a difference between structural dysfunction and functional dysfunction. First, it is important to understand the distinction between a dysfunctional segment and a structural anomaly. A structural anomaly denotes something that can be seen as abnormal on an X-ray or MRI. A structural dysfunction cannot be seen on imaging—it can only be determined by a thorough physical examination with movement testing.

Structural dysfunction refers to problems with the position of a vertebral segment in relation to the rest of the spine; it can then be further categorized as either a positional or motion dysfunction. A positional dysfunction can mean that a vertebra is rotated, flexed, or extended in a static position relative to the vertebra above and below. If this is the case, the vertebral segment will appear out of alignment in a neutral position and will also remain out of alignment during certain movements of the spine (see Figure 2.7).

a. b. c.

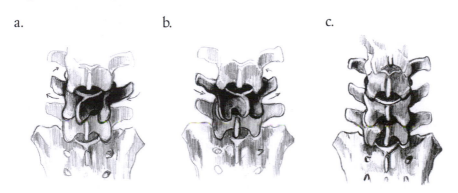

Figure 2.7 Positional dysfunction of L4 vertebrae: a. rotated to the right; b. rotated to the left; c. normal spine

In contrast, when there is a motion dysfunction, the vertebra looks normal in a static position, but there is a limitation of the normal range of motion in the joint, *a limitation that presents itself with movement only*. For example, suppose that a student's *right* facet joint on L4 is stuck in extension, meaning that it cannot move into flexion and, therefore, is restricted or limited in flexion. In spinal extension and in neutral, everything looks normal, but when the student moves into a forward bend, one of the facet joints does not move into flexion. This will cause a rotation of the vertebral segment to the right, affecting the entire kinetic chain of the spine. Everything on an X-ray and/or MRI will appear normal, but the individual may experience symptoms due to this motion dysfunction. Such symptoms would most likely be present with lumbar flexion, as that is where the motion dysfunction is most prominent (see Figure 2.8 a.).

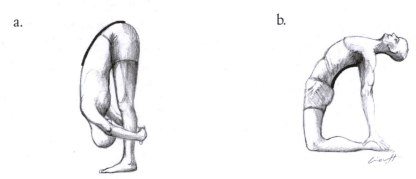

a.   b.

Figure 2.8 Motion dysfunction—appears normal in neutral but: a. rotates to the right with lumbar flexion (due to the right facet joint stuck in extension); b. rotates to the right in lumbar extension (due to the left facet joint stuck in flexion)

A second possibility is that the facet joint on the *left* of the L4 vertebral segment is stuck in flexion. That means that every time an individual moves into spinal extension, the left facet joint cannot glide backwards into extension and it remains in a flexed position. This also causes a right rotation of the vertebral segment, but only when the spine moves into extension. In this case, it is likely that the individual would experience symptoms of discomfort mostly when in back bends, as the spine would appear to be—and would feel—normal in neutral and in forward bends (see Figure 2.8 b.).

Let's explore this concept of motion dysfunction a little more deeply within the practice of yoga. If your student has a dysfunction in which the facet joint is stuck in flexion (as above), this student would feel good when in neutral, as in Tadasana and during all forward bends. She may find that she often gravitates towards forward bending in general to relieve any discomfort. She would experience discomfort or pain in poses like Bhujangasana (cobra),

Ustrasana (camel), Urdvah Mukha Svanasana (upward-facing dog), and most other back bends. She may also experience pain when twisting to the left, as that movement requires a backwards glide of the left facet joint (which in her case is the limited side). Twisting to the right would be pain-free, since the left facet joint only needs to move into flexion and it is already stuck in that position.

In contrast to such structural and movement dysfunctions, an individual can have a *functional dysfunction*, which means a difficulty or inability to recruit the proper muscles in the correct order needed in order to accomplish a specific movement. These faulty movement patterns become habits ingrained in the neuromuscular system and can only be changed with persistent corrective practice, such as we do in yoga. The key is repetition, repetition, repetition! If your student falls into this category, neither diagnostic imaging nor a static examination of the spine and surrounding structures will show any abnormality. You will need to observe the student or client's movement patterns and analyze where and why certain habits and muscular patterns are creating pain and dysfunction. In order to do this, you will also need to develop your ability to skillfully observe and read bodies, in addition to gaining a solid understanding of anatomy and normal biomechanics. When working with yoga practitioners, it is important not only to observe their physical postures, but also to look at them as they move through their yoga asana, their transitions between the postures, and also while they walk, sit, and stand. You can gather a great deal of information about the source(s) of their pain by using this method of evaluation.

PRACTICE TIP 6

FUNCTIONAL DYSFUNCTION SCAN

In order to determine whether your student has a pattern of movement that may be contributing to pain and/or discomfort, it is important to observe him or her in various positions. You might try these suggestions:

- In standing, have the student or client roll forward, vertebra by vertebra, into a forward bend. Notice if there's a shift to one side as they lower down or rise back up. Is there a point where the person stops or do they move fluidly through the range of motion?

- Watch the person walk from the back and from the front. You can tell a great deal about their tendencies by their gait pattern. Do they lean to one side more than the other? Is there movement in the pelvis? In the trunk? What are the arms doing? Where is the head? Is the step length the same on both sides or is there asymmetry?

- Assess your students with yoga postures that they are comfortable with, and observe how they come into and get out of each pose, in addition to their alignment. Try three to five main poses, including poses in which the spine is in neutral, flexion, extension, lateral bending, and rotation.

- Observe your students during functional movements that are common for them throughout the day. Perhaps you will want to watch them at their workstation, or simulating positions they are required to be in at work. Ask them to show you what they do for many hours a day and observe their tendencies in these activities. Make sure not to correct. At this stage you want to observe and notice where clinical symptoms may coincide with certain patterns of movement that may be creating extra loading for their spine. Document your findings at the end of the spinal screening form (see Figure 2.9).

The red herring–getting to the source

Just possibly, when you think you have the reason for the pain all figured out, you might need to remind yourself of one more important thing. The source of the problem may be in a completely different area from the one that is experiencing the pain. For example, restricted mobility (hypomobility) or a structural dysfunction at one level can create too much movement (hypermobility) at segments above and below the affected level. So if L4 is the level that is limited and is rotated to the right, as in our example above, this may cause excessive mobility in L5–S1, as that area needs to compensate for the lack of mobility one segment higher. One can go through life with these minor asymmetries, but at some point the wear and tear on L5–S1 may be too much, and that is where injury will occur. This may occur more readily in individuals who challenge their spine by taking it into more extreme ranges of motion, as dancers, athletes, and some yoga practitioners do. Another common area where we see this red herring present itself is with the sacroiliac joint, which we will explore in detail in Chapter 5. Very often a student will present with pain on the right side, and when I complete my evaluation, I find that the problem is that the left side is not moving properly. The side that I work on mobilizing is the left, even if the pain is on the right, because the lack of mobility on the left causes hypermobility on the right. This hypermobility eventually creates a repetitive stress injury, inflammation, and pain. Unless the side that is stuck is treated, anti-inflammatory medication and treatment of the right side will be in vain.

Spinal screening form

So how do we, as yoga teachers or therapists, effectively evaluate the spine? If the task seems overwhelming and complicated, then you are on the right track. My colleague Nicole Mullins and I have developed a spinal screening form that will make that evaluation a bit easier for you (see Figure 2.9). The form provides a framework to help you to evaluate the physical body of individuals experiencing back pain. But before evaluating and working with any student or client, it is important to remember that, as a yoga teacher or therapist, you are not taking on the role of physical therapist, psychotherapist, or medical doctor, but rather, you are evaluating your students or clients by using all the tools that the multifaceted practices of yoga can offer, along with the intuitive wisdom that can only come from your own devotion to your personal practice. For this reason it is essential that you, the practitioner, remain committed to your own self-exploration, personal growth, and evolution, while also maintaining adequate self-care. If you do not take care of your own needs, while maintaining your own sense of balance and your deep connection to your core Truth, how will you be able to show up and remain fully present for your students and clients?

At this point I will work step by step through the screening form that we developed, helping you understand how you can use the results with your clients.

Note: This is a general physical examination/scan to assist the yoga therapist gain a deeper understanding of which tools of yoga to apply to the individual. It is not intended to replace a thorough examination by a healthcare provider or licensed health professional.

Name:

Chief complaint:

Brief history of onset of injury:

Location/quality of pain:

Pain scale (1–10):

Radiating symptoms?   Y   N   Explain

Symptom behavior: (Note whether worse or better in…)

a.m.   p.m.

sitting   standing

rest   activity

constant   intermittent

Constant pain with no relief—refer to professional.

Relevant past medical history:

HTN   Glaucoma   Recent eye surgery

Other:

Medications: (list)

Postural deviations:

Forward head posture	Y	N	
Anterior pelvic tilt	Y	N	
Posterior pelvic tilt	Y	N	
Pelvic asymmetry	Left	Right	None

Leg length discrepancy

Scoliosis (describe)

Segmental forward roll (standing)

Rib hump	Left	Right	None
Lateral deviation	Left	Right	None

Movement testing checklist

Scan and circle:
(L = Limitation, P = Pain, N = Normal)

Forward flexion	L	P	N
Extension	L	P	N
Left lateral flexion	L	P	N
Right lateral flexion	L	P	N
Rotation right	L	P	N
Rotation left	L	P	N

Neuromuscular/strength testing

Heel walk	+	−
Toe walk	+	−
1 big toe extension	+	−

March Test *indicates hypomobility in sacroiliac joint, balance*

Right	+	−
Left	+	−

Red flags—Important questions to ask:

Do you have any weakness in your legs (not due to a previous injury)?   Y   N

Is it progressive?   Y   N

Uncontrolled bowel/bladder   Y   N

Numbness in saddle area   Y   N

Spinal curves: *(D = Decreased, N = Normal, I = Increased)*

Cervical lordosis   D   N   I

Thoracic kyphosis   D   N   I

Lumbar lordosis   D   N   I

Vertebral Compression Test:
Stable/unstable:
Explanation:

Hip mobility assessment:
Hip series (asymmetry/range of movement/limitations):

Straight Leg Raise: Left   Right

Observation of gait, yoga postures, and mobility:

Major findings:

Therapeutic yoga program:

Name _____   Date _____

Figure 2.9 Yoga therapy for the lower back—screening form

1. History

Most of the important information that you will gather will come from listening to your client's story. Begin by finding out what their main complaint is, and then ask what the treatment goal is. Very often we think that the client's goal is to get rid of the pain, but when you truly listen, you may learn that the main goal is to be able to accomplish certain activities that give joy, such as picking up their grandchildren or taking a morning walk by the sea. Maybe their goal from treatment is to be able to sleep through the night without pain. You really need to let your students speak, and listen to what their actual goals are before you move forward with your own agenda. Tailor your sessions to their goals, not yours. Watch your ego and your tendency to want to solve their problems. Instead, see if you can help them to accomplish their goals, which may cause you to change your treatment plan accordingly.

Take a current history, including the location of the pain, onset, duration, frequency, and nature of symptoms. Start to notice whether the symptoms indicate a spondylogenic type of pain (relating to the facet joints in the spine) radicular pain (nerve root compression), or sacroiliac joint pain (see chart below).

SPONDYLOGENIC	RADICULAR	SACROILIAC JOINT
Diffuse, aching pain	Sharp, burning pain	Sharp pain over SI joint (can radiate to groin area)
Negative straight leg raise (SLR)	Positive SLR	Negative SLR
No sensation changes	Change of sensation related to nerve distribution (dermatomes)	No sensation changes
No weakness in legs	Weakness in areas related to nerve distribution	No weakness in legs
No change in reflexes	Change in reflexes	No change in reflexes
Worse with flexion or extension	Worse with forward flexion	Worse with flexion or extension

Adapted from Ellis (2006)

Be sure also to take note of the student or patient's past medical history. Find out what medications they are taking and if there is any link between past illnesses or accidents and their current complaint. Determine whether they have hypertension or glaucoma, or had recent eye surgery, as those are contraindicated for practicing inversions, and for using the yoga wall for traction.

Note: Even if someone is on medication for hypertension, that person cannot invert, as the medication controls the blood pressure and the body cannot regulate it on its own. So: no inversions even if someone is on high blood pressure medication!

Make sure to ask if there have been any other muscular or neuromuscular diseases in the past as those will affect your examination results. For example, if someone had polio as a child, that person may still have weakness in one leg. If you are evaluating them and find this weakness, you may assume they have a disc herniation at a certain level that corresponds to their weakness while, in fact, the weakness has been there since childhood.

2. Red flags

As you continue to listen to their story, begin to notice if any "red flags" pop up. Any progressive numbness or weakness, saddle area anesthesia (numbness in the pelvic floor area and anus), and bowel and bladder problems can indicate a more serious condition. You should not hesitate to refer your client to a medical professional to clear up any doubt about a more serious condition that may require medical attention. One of the most important signs of a serious condition that may not be mechanical in nature is constant pain with no relief. If your student complains of pain that does not fit a particular pattern or movement, and if he does not find any relief with different positioning or exercises, have him see a medical doctor to clear treatment with you. There are a few conditions, including tumors and systemic problems, that can mimic generalized back pain. When in doubt, it is better to be safe than sorry. Without causing alarm, recommend that your client see a professional to ensure that yoga therapy is indicated and appropriate for them at this time.

3. Observation/postural screening

Soon after taking a complete history it is important to begin the physical examination. You should already have a sense of what may be going on, based on the information you have gathered. Now you need to check if the physical exam confirms your hypothesis so that you can build a picture of what is really happening in the body. Start by observing your client's posture from the front, back, and side. Notice the quality of the curves of the spine, and which ones are increased or decreased. Can you observe an obvious scoliotic curve (an S curve) from the back? Look at the quality of the musculature surrounding the curves. Is there an area that seems more prominent? Sometimes you can see which muscles are working harder than others in order to compensate for faulty alignment. Note these findings.

Vertebral Compression Test

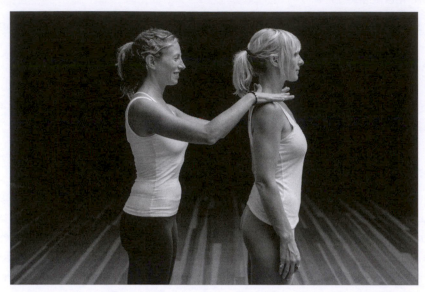

Figure 2.10 Vertebral Compression Test

This test will let you know where the weakest link in the spine is. Stand behind your client and apply downward pressure on their shoulders at a 90° angle. If the spine is stacked correctly, the spine should be stable and there will be no movement in the trunk. However, if there is any postural misalignment, the trunk will collapse in the direction in which the spine bears the weight of gravity. Then provide instructions to your client to help correct their posture—in other words, bring them into Tadasana (mountain pose) for *their* body. Retest and see whether the adjustments you made create more stability in the spine. If so, have your client practice these adjustments at home to improve their postural alignment.

Next, list any obvious postural deviations. Forward head posture refers to the head jutting forward, causing the lower cervical spine to be in flexion and the upper cervical spine to be in extension. This is a common posture that can result when clients work on a computer for hours each day, as well as when they look down at their smart phones. I have been noticing more and more that my clients are experiencing back and neck pain due to the loss of the natural cervical curve caused by their constant staring at current technology. Lower back pain used to be the most common condition in my clinic, but it seems now that upper back and neck pain is beginning to emerge as a more frequent complaint.

Another easy-to-spot postural deviation is sway back, which refers to an excessive lumbar curve. This usually presents itself along with the client's tendency to push the hips forward and externally rotate the legs—movements that create tightness in the hamstrings and the external rotators in the hip. Sway back is also indicative of weakness in the abdominals and pelvic floor, as well as increased compression in the lumbar spine. Look at the pelvis and note if it is tilted anteriorly or posteriorly in standing. An *anterior* tilt is indicative of tightness in the hip flexors, so it would help to work on stretches for this area, especially the iliopsoas muscle. A *posterior* tilt indicates tightness in the hamstring muscles. Check to see if the iliac crest is level on both sides of the pelvis. Does the patient hike one hip higher than the other? Sometimes a scoliotic curve is due to pelvic asymmetry. Pelvic asymmetry can indicate that the quadratus lumborum muscle (which connects the lumbar vertebrae to the pelvis) may be tighter on one side, causing imbalance. Another cause for asymmetry can be a leg length discrepancy. It is important to assess for this with the client in a lying down position, and also sitting against a wall with both legs extended, as in Dandasana (staff pose). You will need to distinguish between a true leg length discrepancy and the *appearance* of one leg being longer than the other due to tightness in the muscles or a rotational component in the pelvis. Very often individuals are told they have one leg longer than the other when, in fact, the appearance of this difference is due to other factors. Such people might be prescribed a heel lift, which actually throws them more off balance than they were in the first place. As Knutson (2005) argues in "Anatomic and functional leg-length inequality: A review and recommendation for clinical decision-making," in general, most people do not need a heel lift even in the case of a leg length discrepancy, unless the difference between the legs is greater than three-quarters of an inch (2cm).

4. Movement testing and special tests

Continuing to paint a full picture of your client, you need to explore his or her range of motion as well as quality of movement. Both are important to observe, as someone can have full range of motion but may also have developed strategies of movement that contribute to their discomfort. In the screening form you will circle whether the range of motion is limited or normal and whether there is pain or not. You can get quite specific here and note the range of movement by degrees or percentage of normal, so that you can re-evaluate down the road and note any progress.

Listed below are several ways that you may ask your client to move to help you diagnose specific structural or movement dysfunctions:

Segmental Rolling

This refers to observing the client as they move into forward flexion vertebra by vertebra, rolling down one spinal segment at a time. Here you can see whether there is a true scoliosis, as one side of the spine or rib cage will be elevated on the convex side of the curve, which will create what is called a "rib hump." You will also want to note if the client deviates to one side while rolling down into flexion, to begin to observe their patterns of movement and neuromuscular sequencing.

Neuromuscular Scan

A nice way to observe lower extremity weakness which can be due to nerve root compression in the lumbar spine is to scan functional movement like walking on the toes and on the heels. In order to walk on the toes, your gastrocnemius muscle needs to be strong enough to lift you up against gravity. The gastrocnemius is innervated by the S1 nerve root, and weakness in this area is indicative of possible nerve root compression in L5–S1. Walking on the heels requires activation of the tibialis anterior muscle, which sits on the lateral side of the anterior shinbone. The nerve that supplies this muscle is the deep peroneal nerve (L4–L5), and any compression at this level will cause the student to have a "drop foot." The muscle that extends the big toe (extensor hallucis longus) is innervated by L4–L5 as well, and any weakness in this area indicates a lesion at this level.

March Test (Gillet's Test)

This is a simple test that can be done to see if there is any sacroiliac joint dysfunction. In truth, evaluating the sacroiliac joint is quite complex and should be done in depth by a licensed physical therapist. The reason this one test is included in the evaluation is to give the yoga therapist a chance to scan this area and note if there is any obvious dysfunction or sacral fixation. It is there to help you continue to solve the mystery. In order to do the March Test, have the patient stand in front of you and place your right thumb on the PSIS (posterior superior iliac spine) while the thumb of your left hand is placed on the sacrum at the same level (see Figure 2.11 a.). The client is asked to lift the right leg off the ground, flexing at the hip higher than 90°. If there is normal movement in the sacroiliac joint, the ipsilateral (same side) pelvis should rotate posteriorly, causing your right thumb to move inferiorly compared to your left thumb. If there is no movement, or if your right thumb actually moves superiorly, this is indicative of a hypomobile sacroiliac joint. You then repeat the test on the left side, placing the left thumb on the PSIS and right thumb on the sacrum at the same level. Ask the patient to flex the left hip and notice if the left PSIS drops or not.

a.

b.

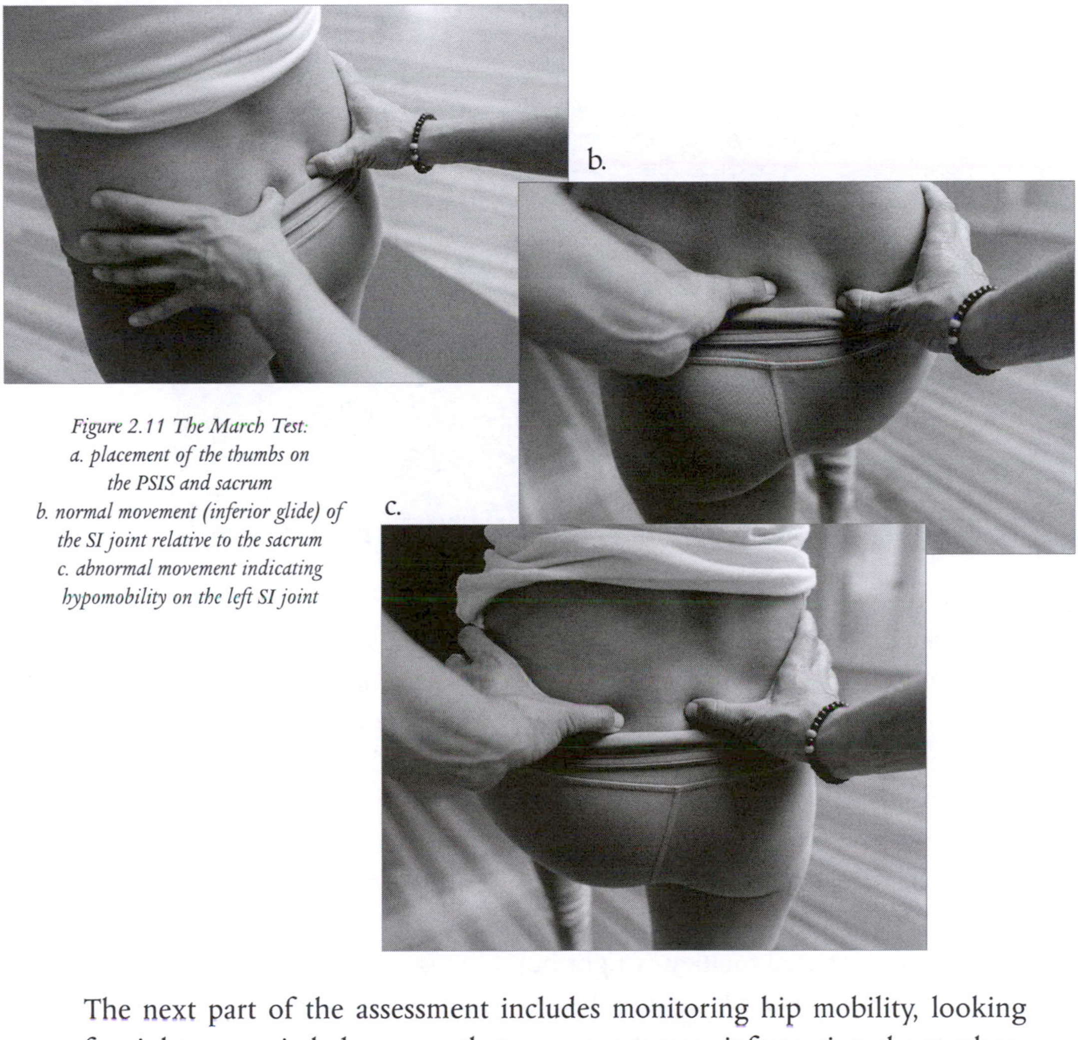

Figure 2.11 The March Test:
a. placement of the thumbs on the PSIS and sacrum
b. normal movement (inferior glide) of the SI joint relative to the sacrum
c. abnormal movement indicating hypomobility on the left SI joint

c.

The next part of the assessment includes monitoring hip mobility, looking for tightness or imbalances so that we can get more information about where to stretch and strengthen. The first test is the Thomas Test, which tests for tightness in the hip flexors.

The Thomas Test

You will need a high table to accomplish this test effectively. Ask your student to sit at the very edge of the table and hug one knee into her chest. She must keep the knee glued to her belly throughout the movement. She then lies back (you can help guide her onto her back), allowing the other leg to hang over the edge of the table. A positive test occurs when the bottom leg does not descend fully onto the table. If the leg remains lifted, the hip flexors are tight. If the knee moves out to the side, there is tightness in the iliotibial band as well.

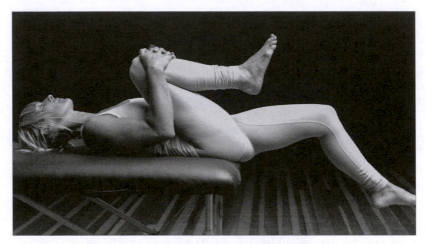

Figure 2.12 The Thomas Test

To gradually release such tightness in the hip flexors, I often prescribe the Purna Yoga Hip Opening Series described in detail in Chapter 4. This is a series of postures that opens the hip in every possible range of motion, along with traction. While it is excellent as a treatment tool, the hip series can also be used as a diagnostic tool to determine where there is imbalance in the body. Look through that section of Chapter 4, and as part of your evaluation ask the student to go through the hip series. Observe carefully and try to notice if one or more movements seem more restricted than the others—for example, external rotation is tight but there is good hamstring flexibility. Make a note of obvious imbalances between various movements. Next, note the differences between the right and left leg. Is there more internal rotation on the right than the left? Which of the quadriceps is tighter in Eka Pada Supta Virasana (hip extension)? The imbalances between right and left sides can also give you a sense of where to work, and of where the source of the problem might be.

Straight Leg Raise

This is a common test used to diagnose a disc herniation or neural tension on the sciatic nerve. The patient lies supine while you lift the leg with the knee straight. A positive test is indicated by sciatic pain when the leg is lifted 30–70°. Symptoms may be exacerbated by flexing the cervical spine, as that movement puts increased tension on the dura.

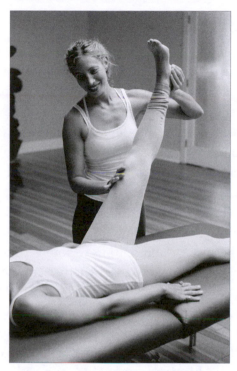

Figure 2.13 The Straight Leg Raise (SLR) Test

Finally, it is essential to observe your student's gait pattern and overall functional mobility. Notice how they walk into your office and how they stand or sit when they are speaking with you. It is best to catch them off guard and notice their inherent patterns of movement that may be contributing to the cause of their lower back pain. I highly recommend reading *Walk Yourself Well* by physical therapist Sherry Brourman (1998/2007). It is a wonderful resource that can help you learn how to assess gait and decide which exercises to prescribe for your students. If your client is a yoga practitioner, it will be important to look at their practice and notice their alignment in the postures. While yoga can be a tool for healing back pain, it can also be the cause if not practiced correctly.

Unfortunately, I learned this lesson firsthand after herniating a disc during a yoga class due to a vigorous practice without adequate integrity. While my injury set me on a path towards a more mindful practice and I am grateful for the insight, this is something we want to avoid for our students. Observe postures that your clients practice, and take notes. Work on modifying their practice accordingly, so as not to re-injure themselves. In addition, you can use certain postures as corrective exercises during their healing process.

Interpreting your findings

After completing the physical evaluation, you should have a good idea in which direction to take your patient in terms of their practice. From the physical evaluation you should have a sense of where the problem is coming from. Is there, for instance, a possible disc herniation, structural or functional dysfunction in the facet joints of the lumbar spine, or a possible sacroiliac joint dysfunction? You can also see which muscles are tight and which are weak and create a plan pinpointing the muscles you want to stretch and/or strengthen. Then you can design a program based on the specific information in the chapters that follow.

Please note that this spinal screening only covers the physical layer of the body. While taking the history and getting to know your student or client during treatment, you will begin to sense whether and what issues may be lodged in the mental, energetic, emotional, and intellectual layers as well.

In my clinic, we have begun incorporating a second assessment tool that addresses those other layers. Developed by TriYoga in Boston, Massachusetts, this form can be filled out by the patient before coming in or during the first visit. Because it is a checklist, it does not take long and gives quite a bit of information about where your patient stands. Also, scanning the answers on the form may lead you to ask questions that may not have come up previously. I will often take a look at something a client wrote and ask him or her to explain more about that section. This opens the conversation up for deeper and more honest exploration.

The TriYoga Total Health Assessment form can help you determine in which of the koshas there are deficits and then design a treatment plan accordingly. In addition, you can use this as a re-evaluation tool so that you can have a more objective measure of your client's quality of life and the effectiveness of your treatment protocol.

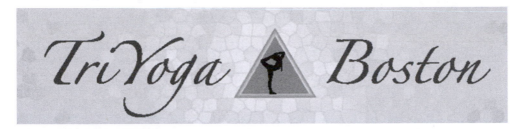

Total Health Assessment

Please note that all information from this assessment will be kept confidential

Student's name: _____

Please check the box that best describes your physical health in the past month.

PHYSICAL BODY	POOR	NEEDS IMPROVEMENT	AVERAGE	GOOD	EXCELLENT
General health					
Physical fitness					
Strength					
Stamina					
Flexibility					
Range of motion					
Endurance					
Balance					
Nutrition					
Digestion					
Elimination					
Exercise habits					
Sleep quality					
Pain control					

Please describe any physical concerns/issues: _____

_____

Please check the box that best describes cognitive/emotional well-being in the past month.

SUBTLE BODY	POOR	NEEDS IMPROVEMENT	AVERAGE	GOOD	EXCELLENT
Breathing					
Energy level					
Mood					

POSITIVE COGNITIVE AND EMOTIONAL QUALITIES	NEVER	ALMOST NEVER	OCCASIONALLY	USUALLY	ALWAYS
Feel hopeful about the future					
Feel contented					
Feel calm					
Feel relaxed					
Feel focused					
Have a good sense of humor					
Acknowledge feelings					
Express feelings appropriately					
Practice forgiveness					
Practice gratitude					

CONCERNS ABOUT COGNITIVE AND EMOTIONAL WELL-BEING	ALWAYS	USUALLY	OCCASIONALLY	ALMOST NEVER	NEVER
Feel worried					
Feel regretful					
Difficulty concentrating					
Feel anxious					
Feel sad					
Feel depressed					
Feel stressed					
Memory difficulties					
Feel angry					

Please describe any cognitive and emotional concerns: _____

_____

Please check the box that best describes your relationships in the past month.

RELATIONSHIPS/ EMOTIONAL WELL-BEING	STRONGLY DISAGREE	DISAGREE	NEUTRAL	AGREE	STRONGLY AGREE
Have people I trust and can go to for support					
Able to make and maintain friendships					
Have close/intimate relationships					
Express love/ concern to those I care about					
I feel comfortable with my sexuality					

Please describe concerns about relationships: _____

_____

_____

Please check the box that best describes your perceptions in the past month:

INTELLECT/ INNER GUIDANCE/ PERCEPTION	STRONGLY DISAGREE	DISAGREE	NEUTRAL	AGREE	STRONGLY AGREE
I have self-awareness of thoughts and feelings					
I listen to my inner voice					
I can observe thoughts and feelings without attachment					
I am sensitive to the feelings of others					
I feel compassion for myself and others					
I am intuitive					
I live mindfully					

Please describe perceptual concerns/issues: _____

_____

_____

Please check the box that best describes your outlook in the past month.

CAUSAL BODY

LIFE SATISFACTION	STRONGLY DISAGREE	DISAGREE	NEUTRAL	AGREE	STRONGLY AGREE
I balance work, school, family, self					
I make time for leisure pursuits					
I am able to set and follow goal(s) for myself					
I feel good about myself					
I am happy with my life					

Life satisfaction perceptual concerns/issues: _____

_____

_____

Please check the box that best describes your spirituality in the past month.

SPIRITUALITY	STRONGLY DISAGREE	DISAGREE	NEUTRAL	AGREE	STRONGLY AGREE
My life has meaning and purpose					
I look forward to growing and changing					
I feel connected to something greater than myself					
I have a spiritual or religious practice					
I make time for self-reflection (affirmations, prayers, meditation)					
I have a vision for my life					
I wish to give back for all that is good in my life					

Spiritual concerns/issues: _____

_____

_____

CASE STUDY:
MARK'S INITIAL EVALUATION

Findings and interpretations

After hearing Mark's story, it was time to begin the physical assessment. He came in with a diagnosis based on his MRI but we still need to see where his functional limitations are. We heard some of his history at the end of Chapter 1, and now here is the information we were able to gather using the spinal assessment.

Mark has more pain in sitting, which is required for his job. His pain is worse in the morning and with bending forward, and feels better when he is at rest on his back with his knees bent. His pain also lessens when he is standing. The pain does radiate down his right leg and he has some decreased sensation over the top of his right foot and heel. He has some weakness in his right toe extensor, extensor hallucis longus (EHL), that has been stable since the injury. He has no bowel or bladder problems, no red flags, no hypertension, and no prior history that is of concern.

Mark's pain seems radicular in nature, as there is pressure on the right sciatic nerve. This indicates the need for spinal traction and decompression in order to decrease pain and restore mobility.

On observation, we can see that Mark has a decreased lumbar curve and that his pelvis sits in a posterior tilt. He also has a forward head posture, mostly due to working at a computer for much of his adult life. He does not exhibit any pelvic asymmetry. If anything, he seems to have decreased mobility in his sacroiliac joint. Observing his gait, we see that there is very little movement in both the pelvis and trunk; he walks as if his limbs were detached from the rest of his torso.

On movement testing, we find that Mark shifts to the left when he bends forward and that his forward bends are limited and painful. His back bends are painful, as well as rotation to the right. All other movements were within normal limits and there is no pelvic asymmetry or leg length discrepancy.

The March Test was negative for SI involvement, but the Straight Leg Raise (SLR) Test was positive on the right for neural tension. In addition, through the hip series, we were able to see that his hamstrings were extremely limited (to about 50° SLR bilaterally), and internal rotation was limited on both sides as well. The Thomas Test was positive for tightness in the hip flexors, and also iliotibial band tightness.

From these findings, we can deduce that Mark's pain is radicular in nature and that it is directly related to his activities of daily living (prolonged sitting and staring at a computer screen), deconditioning, and tightness in the hips.

From observing Mark's answers on the TriYoga evaluation form it was clear that several koshas were out of balance in addition to his physical layer. Most of the imbalances lay in the realm of the cognitive/emotional layer and subtle body. He felt anxious and depressed a great deal of the time and was not fulfilled by his work. Though he had very positive relationships and support, he often felt lonely and unhappy with his life. He longed to feel connected to something deeper. He felt constant internal "tension" and did not feel that he was able to balance family, work, and relationships in a way that gave him personal satisfaction.

After reading the TriYoga form I was able to talk to Mark, who was quite private about his personal life, about things that created this sense of anxiety and depression. He began to open up about painful experiences in his job and in his relationship and about how this back injury really terrified him. I listened carefully, without judgment, and assured him that I would help him with these struggles in addition to the physical problem by using a yoga-based approach.

When he left that day, Mark looked much more relaxed. "I have not been able to tell this to anyone so far, and while it is hard, I feel a lot better now." I smiled at him and thanked him for his openness and honesty.

CHAPTER 3

When it Really Hurts

Relieving Acute Back Pain

Relax your toes.
What have they ever done to you?

Judith Hanson Lasater

When I first started practicing yoga, I wanted to be the best. The more intense the asana class, the better. I couldn't sit still for even a few minutes. What I found was, the harder I worked and the more I moved, the more I could finally relax into Savasana. I tried a few restorative classes but I found them to be boring and considered them to be a waste of time. I wasn't "doing" anything. Unless I could feel the sweat and the burn, I felt that nothing was happening.

Still, this was a valuable time. My yoga practice was a way to work so hard physically that any stresses, anxieties, and deep disappointments I had been feeling were momentarily forgotten, and I had no choice but to be present in my body. What this precious time gave me was the feeling of what it could be like if my mind were quiet for just an hour. It showed me a glimpse of another reality that I could access.

Surely you have noticed this in your students or clients, the sense of release, peace, and even bliss they experience towards the end of a session. Once I injured my back, I was unable to practice as I had previously, yet I still craved the respite from my over-analytical and busy mind. I decided to begin practicing Iyengar Yoga because it was alignment-based and the teachers were able to modify poses for my condition. Because Iyengar is a slower, more methodical practice, often with longer holds, I now had to focus on the details of my asana instead of "powering" through the poses. I was asked to feel the sensations in my body and respond to them. I was forced to be still just long enough to start to see what was really going on inside. And what I saw was not always pretty.

Most of us push forward in life at an incredible pace, racing from one activity, one job, and one social engagement to another. We are overstimulated

79

by constant information jumping out at us from email, texts, and voicemail in devices that we carry with us all the time. If we are not "doing" something, society tells us that we are lazy and unproductive. To add insult to injury, many of us must also deal with our own inner critics telling us how we will never be good enough and have to work harder, or be better, to deserve love and acceptance.

Then, we go to yoga class to "relax." But what we tend to do is push ourselves to excel just as we do in the outside world. A physically vigorous practice is good, especially when we have a sedentary life; but it also needs to be balanced with a more reflective and grounding practice so we are not always on fast speed. Slowing down may prove one of the greatest challenges for your students, and perhaps for you as well.

To my surprise, my home practice has become slow and gentle lately. So much so, that I sometimes wonder if I am just being lazy. Then I remind myself of the intensity of life around me, and all that I do each day: seeing patients, teaching classes and workshops, writing, managing a clinic, and being a single mom. And then it hits me that slow and gentle are probably just what I need. Time to be kind to myself. Time to focus on my breath and calm my nervous system. Time to focus on my feet on the ground and to allow my whirling mind to settle and soften. Time to let go—of the holding, gripping, and striving. Time to just be.

If your students practice yoga with aggression, they will only create more tension in body and mind. When they do not stop and listen to the messages being sent by their bodies, and instead continue pushing forward, then they develop injuries. It is not the yoga that creates injuries, but rather the *way* it is practiced that can cause harm. The solution for them is to *slow down, pay attention, and be kind* to themselves. That is how true healing happens.

Yoga is about balance; it is the middle way. Yoga is about practicing the strong poses with greater relaxation and the relaxing postures with more focused awareness. It is about knowing what you need on any given day and adapting your practice to your emotional, mental, and physical state. Like ocean swimming, yoga asks us to explore the unknowns of the deep within us, and in the process cleanse and heal ourselves, and become more self-aware.

When, for instance, your students or clients are dealing with back pain, they must learn to let go of the tension in the spinal muscles before any specific changes can be made. The muscles surrounding the spine will go into spasm and clamp down whenever there is any injury or dysfunction in the body. This is a protective mechanism designed to prevent any further injury to the spine. For an acute injury, this type of muscle tension is appropriate; however, many of those you instruct will be operating in a constant state of internal spasm or "gripping." Until this tightness can be released, it will

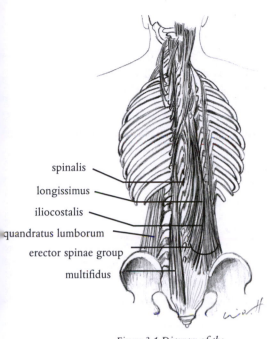

spinalis

longissimus

iliocostalis

quandratus lumborum

erector spinae group

multifidus

*Figure 3.1 Diagram of the
deep muscles of the spine*

be difficult for you to help them correct the dysfunction that caused the muscles to spasm in the first place.

The deep muscles around the spine become tight with injury, but they also tighten up as a response to stress and inner tension. Our bodies are mirrors of our internal worlds. When there is a sense of lack of control in life, or fear, our deep spinal muscles respond accordingly. In *Healing Back Pain* (1991), John Sarno discusses the emotional landscape of individuals who experience back discomfort. He states that these are generally individuals who create a great deal of internal pressure to succeed. They may be calm on the outside, but a bundle of nerves on the inside. They are always working hard, trying to be better, slowly building up pressure to prove themselves personally and professionally. Sarno argues that such pain is due not to structural abnormalities but to a condition called "tension myositis syndrome" (TMS), which is a result of emotional tension and anxiety and occurs most often between the ages of 30 and 60, the years when there is the most responsibility and pressure to excel and succeed.

From a yogic perspective, Aadil Palkhivala teaches that the lower back is linked with the root chakra, the energy center at the base of the spine, which symbolizes our concept of safety and security. The sacrum and lower back are the seat of survival, and respond to stresses involving money, power, and sex. If people feel unsupported in their lives, then it makes sense that pain will manifest in the place that bears the weight of the world—the L5–S1 junction. If such people are lucky, they have already found you. Here is a tip you can give them, to learn how to breathe into the tense places.

PRACTICE TIP 7

Stand in mountain pose for a moment. Close your eyes. Begin to notice where you are holding tension in your body. Often we hold tension in the following areas: the buttocks, the lower back, the upper trapezius, the jaw, and the forehead. Notice your breath. Is it shallow and tense? See if you can take a deep breath moving the air into your primary area of tension, and then release the tension from that muscle group on the exhalation. Repeat five times. Notice that you can relax a specific part of your body by moving your breath and awareness into that area.

Acute lower back pain program

For the first few weeks following an injury, especially an acute disc bulge or herniation, there will be a great deal of muscle spasm and pain. In the early phases treatment will focus on careful positioning, as well as some of the anti-inflammatory treatments offered by Ayurveda, the sister science of yoga. Once the initial spasm calms down, you can begin guiding your client or student toward more movement and yoga postures. Then come exercises that involve gentle traction, while you also help them to increase their postural awareness in order to change any habits that create dysfunction, misalignment, or strain in standing and sitting.

Proper positioning

90/90: Instruct your student or client to begin lying on their back with legs elevated and calves resting on a chair or couch at a 90° angle. Have them hold this position for 15 minutes. They can also lie on an ice pack or bag of frozen peas placed under the sacrum in this position.

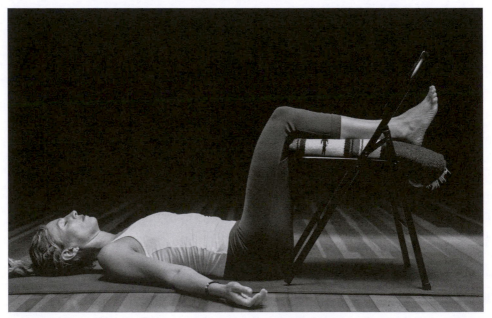

Figure 3.2 Position 90/90 for acute back pain

Extended child's pose/Forward Virasana

Have your client spread the knees wide with the toes touching. Ask them to stretch out through the fingertips, keeping the elbows and wrists off the floor (Figure 3.3 a.). Then they should push the floor away from themselves with the fingertips, while bringing the hips back onto the heels in order to lengthen the spine. Invite them to spread the shoulder blades wide on the back. As they inhale, tell them to invite the breath into the spine; as they exhale, tell them to focus on releasing tension in that area. The hold should last one to two minutes.

Modifications: If the head doesn't touch the floor, place a block or blanket under the forehead. If the client has knee problems or decreased knee flexion, place a folded blanket in the knee crease and support the head with a block or blanket (Figure 3.3 b.). If tight ankles are an issue, place a folded blanket under the knees and ankle joints, allowing the feet to come off the blanket (Figure 3.3 c.). This makes space for the ankle joint to stretch into plantar flexion without pain. If there is any pain in the knees, omit this posture.

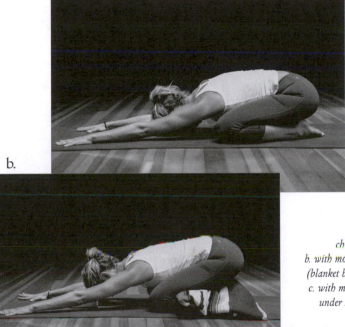

Figure 3.3 a. Extended
child's pose / Forward Virasana
b. with modification for decreased knee flexion
(blanket between knees and block under head)
c. with modification for tight ankles (blanket
under shins, tops of feet off the blanket)

Knees to chest

Invite your client to lie on his back and hug the knees into the chest. As the knees move in towards the chest, ask him to deepen the groin and feel the tailbone moving away from the head. The idea is to feel the lower back lengthening on the floor as the knees move in towards the chest so as to keep the sacrum in contact with the earth. Hold for five minutes.

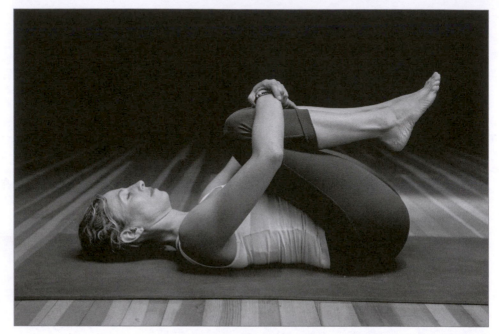

Figure 3.4 Knees to chest

Prone to baby cobra

This position may be painful for some individuals, while it may feel good for others. This will depend on the type of dysfunction that is occurring in the spine. If this position does aggravate the client's condition, tell her to respect her body's messages and omit this position. The intention is to find what works for each individual.

Invite your client or student to place her hands under her shoulders at the nipple line. Keep the legs hips' distance apart and press all five toes into the earth, *especially the pinky toe side*, to protect her back. Have the client inhale, pulling the floor towards her with her fingertips as she rolls the shoulders back and down. See that she continues to squeeze her elbows into the waist and moves her shoulder blades away from her ears. Have her keep her forehead on the ground initially. Repeat five to ten times as tolerated.

a.

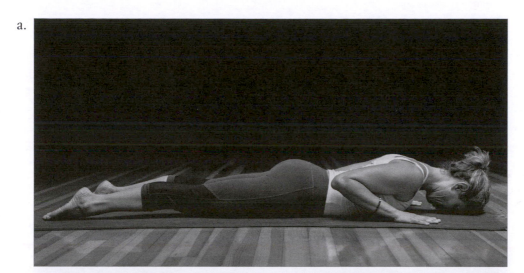

b.

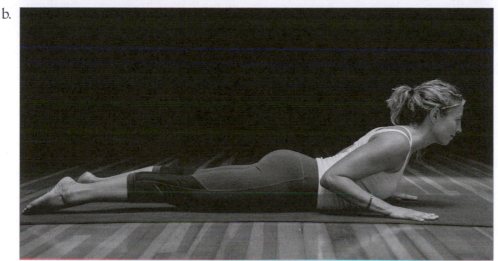

Figure 3.5 a. Prone position; b. baby cobra/Bhujangasana

If it feels good, you can work on having her lift her rib cage off the floor, focusing on lengthening the spine as she moves into extension. Have her imagine her vertebrae as pearls in a necklace. Instead of hinging at one level, work vertebra by vertebra, instructing her to move each one into the body as she lifts.

Have your student imagine that there is a circle above her lower back. As she comes up into spinal extension, instruct her to visualize the center of the circle and begin to move each vertebra away from the radius (see Figure 3.6).

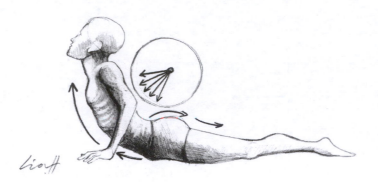

Figure 3.6 Cobra/Bhujangasana using a circle and radius for reference

This technique can be done with manual assistance as well. To aid your student in feeling the vertebrae move into extension, place your fingers on the spinous processes of their L5 vertebra and instruct the student to move the vertebra away from your finger as they exhale. In other words, they will move the spine *into* the body on each exhalation. Continue to move up the spine and provide feedback when you feel the student is able to accomplish this action.

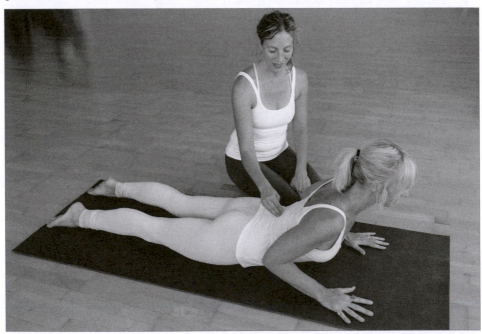

Figure 3.7 Working in pairs to assist extension of each lumbar vertebrae in Bhujangasana (cobra pose)

Anti-inflammatory modalities

Ayurveda, the sister science of yoga, offers many natural and food-related remedies for both acute and ongoing pain. Natural anti-inflammatories include icing the area of pain for 10 to 15 minutes. Turmeric has anti-inflammatory properties and can be taken, either in food or as a supplement, over the long term for best results. You can also recommend an application of Sunbreeze Oil, a Sunrider product (see www.sunrider.com), to the affected area for enhanced pain relief. Rubbing oils such as a product I use in my clinic— Mahavishgarbha Oil by Tattva's Herbs—may help as well, for in its sesame oil base are many herbs that are soothing to inflamed muscle and tissue, which also promote joint health. We want to keep the joints as well lubricated as possible, as dry joints become arthritic. If your students do not have access to this oil, try plain sesame oil; turmeric can be added to it. Encourage them to also eat good fats such as avocado, nuts, coconut oil, and ghee.

You will also want to suggest that they eat a more alkaline diet, as injuries cannot heal in an acidic state. Lots of leafy greens and warm, wet foods such as soups, lentils, and stews are helpful as well. Back pain clients should limit their intake of sugar (especially refined), white flour, coffee, and alcohol, as those add to the dehydration of joints over time.

The treatments that Ayurveda offers to heal acute injury can be summed up by the treatments offered at a clinic in Kerala, India, which specializes in Ayurvedic sports medicine. The Ayurvedic treatments to heal acute injury involve internal medicines, such as herbs and diet; external medicines, such as *lepas* (herbalized pastes) and *patrapinda sveda* (massage with warmed leaves of anti-inflammatory plants); procedures such as *varma chikitsa* to increase joint mobility and function and decrease pain; *pancha karma*, which removes toxins and cleanses the body; and traditional physiotherapy With this holistic approach, Ayurvedic treatment can be a good route to healing and, like therapeutic yoga, an alternative to surgery.

Gentle traction

In the initial phases of the injury we want to be very careful with traction. As mentioned before, the muscles surrounding the spine will spasm as a result of the injury to protect the spine. Sometimes, if practiced too soon or too aggressively, although traction will feel good while it is being applied, the muscles will spasm more when traction is released. That is why it is important to start with gentle traction in a supine position, and progress your clients from shorter to longer holds to make sure there is no backlash.

The techniques listed below describe good, safe positions to offer your clients so they can begin to experience traction in their spines.

1. Finding the pit of the abdomen with a stick

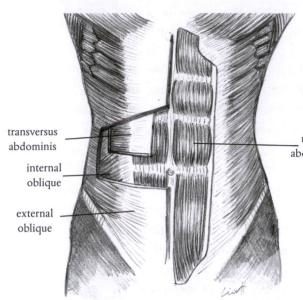

transversus abdominis

internal oblique

external oblique

rectus abdominis

Figure 3.8 Diagram of the pit of the abdomen (POA)

Finding the pit of the abdomen (POA) is one of the key factors to improving back health and achieving long-term pain relief. The POA is the area between the navel and the pubic bone and comprises the transversus abdominis, rectus abdominis, and external and internal obliques.

To find it, have your students lie on their backs and place their hands on their bellies below the navel. Invite them to take a deep inhalation and feel the belly rise, and then exhale, feeling the belly fall under their hands. *On their next exhalation, ask them to draw the lower belly area back towards the spine and up toward the head.* Repeat this action with each exhalation, relaxing the belly on the inhalation.

Sometimes it is difficult for students to wake up this part of the body, especially if they have never engaged their core in this subtle way in the past. In fact, most individuals who experience back pain have never learned how to access this part of the body. Be patient with your students or clients. At first, they may only be thinking about doing it in their heads. But with time and practice, the POA will wake up. And it will change their lives—or at least their yoga practice. On the following page is another tip to share with your students.

2. Auto traction: Gentle unilateral traction for the spine

Invite your students or clients to lie on their backs with knees bent. Have them place the heel of each hand in the hip creases, and then take a deep inhalation. As they exhale, invite them to lift the lower belly towards their heads as they push the right thighbone away from the head. Cue them to inhale as they relax, then to exhale, and lift the POA and push the thighbone away from the head before repeating on the left side.

Repeat nine times on each side, alternating sides for unilateral traction, which is less aggravating to the spine.

PRACTICE TIP 8

To help you find your POA you will need a long rod or stick.

Lie on your back and place a long rod in the area of the POA just beneath the navel area. Rest the other end of it on a wall.

As you inhale, you should see the top of the rod rise against the wall. On the exhalation, imagine drawing the POA in and up towards your head. As you accomplish this action, the rod will serve as a visual cue as it descends over the wall. The pressure of the rod into the POA area will also provide some kinesthetic feedback to the area to help increase awareness and facilitate activation.

Do three sets of ten repetitions. Remove the rod and try it again. You should still be able to sense the rod in the lower belly area as you continue to practice.

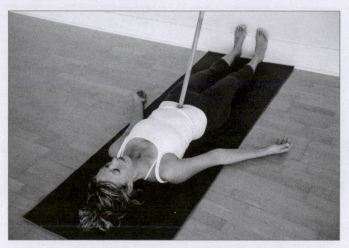

Figure 3.9 Rod placement in the pit of the abdomen (POA)

Next practice lifting the POA in sitting and standing (it is more challenging than the supine position). Then start to incorporate it into your yoga postures.

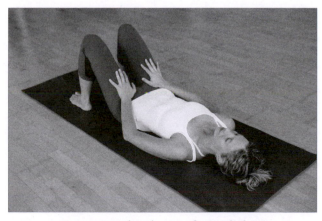

Figure 3.10 Unilateral traction for acute back pain

3. Yoga wall variation

Ask your students to lie supine with feet on the yoga wall (shins parallel to the floor), with the yoga strap in the hip crease. Place blocks in line with their hands against the yoga wall, so that they can press into the blocks with their hands, creating traction in the lower back. Do it one side at a time, while lifting the POA on the same side for unilateral traction. Repeat nine times on each side.

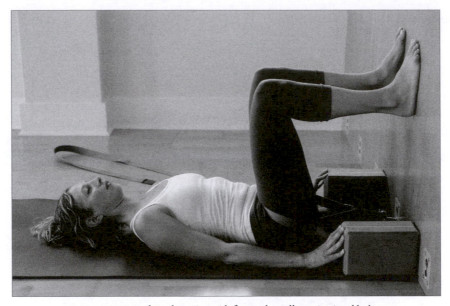

Figure 3.11 Unilateral traction with feet on the wall pressing into blocks

4. Reclining hand to big toe pose/Supta Padangusthasana with traction

For this posture your client or students will need two straps. One strap will be used as a loop to traction the hip joint and the other is to help hold the leg up in the air. Have them place the looped strap in the right hip crease and in the arch of the left foot. Make sure the strap buckle is facing away from the head, so that when they tighten it, it tractions the right hip.

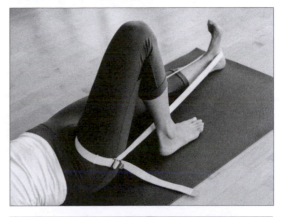

Figure 3.12 Placement of straps for reclining hand to big toe pose/ Supta Padangusthasana in hip crease and opposite heel

Next, instruct them to extend the right leg up towards a 90° angle (Figure 3.13). They should feel the strap securely in the right hip crease, pulling the thighbone away from the head. Next, ask them to press their left foot into the strap, making sure that the toes point straight up. Have them engage the quadriceps, contracting the right quadriceps as well, focusing on moving the right thighbone away from the head. Once again, ask them to lift the POA towards the head, lengthening the lower back. Hold for one to two minutes, and repeat two to three times on each side.

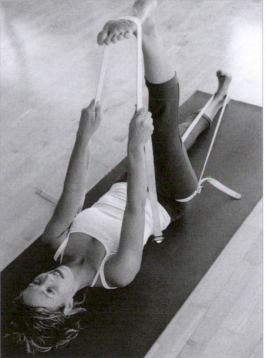

Figure 3.13 Supta Padangusthasana with two straps

5. Self-traction holding onto a bar or with partner

Instruct your client or student to hold onto a wall bar or railing with the hands at shoulder distance, before walking the feet slightly in front of the hips. Have them shift the hips back and feel as if the pelvis is being pulled away from the rib cage. They should keep the shoulders in joint so that the traction occurs in the spine and not in the shoulder joint.

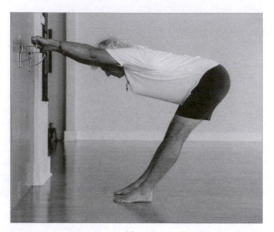

Figure 3.14 Self-traction with a bar

Partner variation: Here, have the client or student place a strap in the hip crease and have a partner lean back (elbows into the waist to protect the lower back) to increase the traction. Guide them always to remember to breathe and relieve tension in the lower back area by bringing mindfulness into this posture.

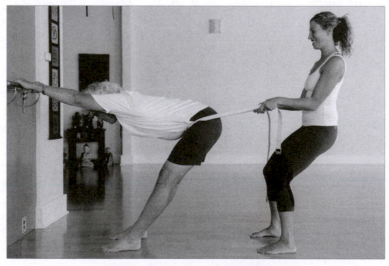

Figure 3.15 Self-traction with a bar and partner

6. Traction on door or yoga wall with cross stretch

Using the yoga wall or traction-on-door set-up with two straps looped together and a block (see Figures 6.5 and 6.6 in Chapter 6), invite the students to walk their heels up the wall as they extend their arms out into downward-facing dog pose. Have them keep the quadriceps engaged, and lengthen throughout the spine. On the exhalation, ask them to bend the right knee and stretch out through the right fingertips while lengthening through the left sitting bone. Next they should inhale and straighten the right knee. On the next exhalation, have them bend the left knee and stretch out through the left fingertips, reaching in the opposite direction with the right sitting bone. Repeat the right- and left-side movements for a minimum of three times. (For more on traction see Chapter 6.)

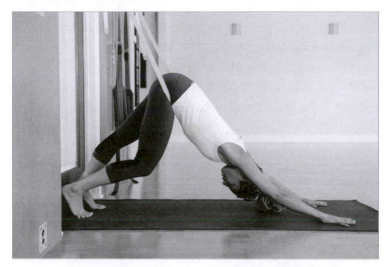

Figure 3.16 Traction on a door with cross stretch

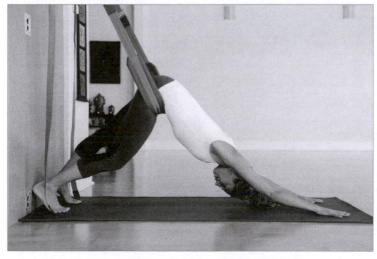

Figure 3.17 Traction on yoga wall with cross stretch

The Purna Yoga Low Back Series

As the pain lessens, this series of postures will afford safe relief. This series was given to my teacher, Aadil Palkhivala, by B.K.S. Iyengar after he sustained multiple disc herniations following a traumatic injury. It is a subtle sequence and safe for most to perform. It is important to have your client or student do these exercises on a yoga mat so that they will not slide easily. This resistance will create the tension necessary to traction the sacrum and lower back area. This sequence will often relieve or reduce pain immediately. If the student has no pain, have them practice standing before doing the sequence, and re-evaluate when they are done. They may notice that it feels easier to stand up tall with less gripping in the lower back and hips after performing this series.

The low back series is an incredible and safe way to release tension in the spine, create traction, and release the hip flexors, all of which are essential for individuals with back pain. It is important to coordinate breath with movement, as all actions occur on the exhalation only.

You will need a yoga mat and a wall, and some individuals will need a strap as well. The series is in three parts; each exercise should be repeated three times, alternating legs. Here I will give you the exact instructions, and you should communicate them in exactly the same way to your client or student.

Part 1

a.

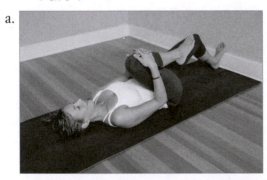

b.

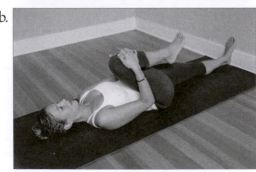

Figure 3.18 Part 1 of low back series: a. starting position; b. ending position

Place your mat perpendicular to the wall. Lie on your back with both feet against the wall and both knees bent at a 45° angle. Make sure your toes are pointed straight up and not turned out to the sides. Then bring the right knee into the chest with both hands (see Figure 3.18 a.).

Inhale deeply. On the exhalation, push into the wall with your left foot and contract the left thigh strongly, pushing yourself away from the wall along the mat (Figure 3.18 b.). Press your lower back into the mat as you slide along the mat. This will help to release tight back muscles.

Keep holding the right knee in towards the chest.

Inhale, release the bottom leg and then the top leg, and wiggle the buttocks towards the wall. This wiggling action is important as it releases and retrains the spinal muscles. Avoid sitting up during this action.

Repeat with the right foot against the wall and the left knee held into the chest. Repeat the right- and left-side movements three times.

Part 2

a.

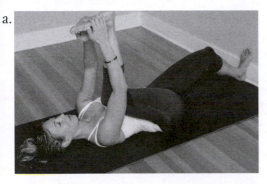

b.

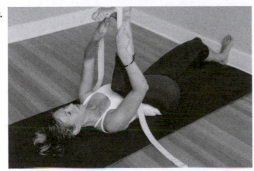

Begin with both feet against the wall and knees bent, as in the first exercise. Bring your right knee towards your chest and grasp both sides of the right foot with both hands as you bring the thigh down towards your chest. The sole of the foot should be parallel with the ceiling and the shin should be perpendicular to the thigh (Figure 3.19 a.); use a strap if necessary (Figure 3.19 b.).

Without moving the right leg, exhale as you push away from the wall with the left leg. Keep the thighbone pressing down to the ground for the duration of the exhalation. Inhaling, relax the bottom leg, then the top leg. Scoot in towards the wall. Repeat on the other side. Repeat the right- and left-side movements three times.

c.

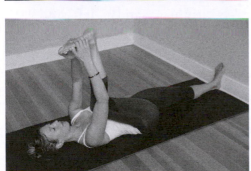

d.

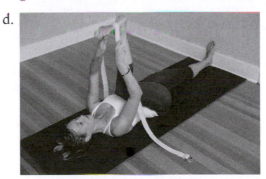

Figure 3.19 Part 2 of the low back series: a. starting position (holding onto foot); b. starting position (with strap); c. ending position (holding onto foot); d. ending position (with strap)

Part 3

a.
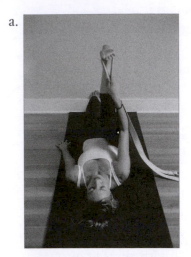

b.
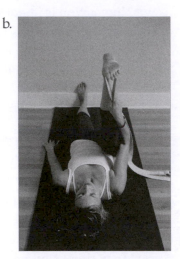

c.
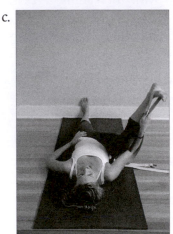

d.
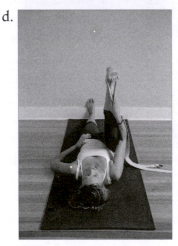

Figure 3.20 Part 3 of low back series: a. starting position; b. push away from the wall; c. bring the leg out to the side; d. bring leg back to center

Repeat the second exercise, holding the upper foot on the outside with one hand, with the forearm supporting the outside of the knee (Figure 3.20 a.). Exhaling, push away from the wall with the opposite leg (Figure 3.20 b.). Take a deep inhalation, and as you exhale, bring the top leg out to the side as far as you can go, while keeping the pelvis level (Figure 3.20 c.). Take one more inhalation. On the next exhalation, bring the leg back to center (Figure 3.20 d.). On the next exhalation, release the legs and scoot in towards the wall. Repeat on the other side. Repeat the right- and left-side movements three times.

To come up, bend both knees and place both feet on the floor. Roll to the side and push up to a standing position. Avoid sitting up abruptly, as this will cause your psoas muscle to contract, which will decrease the benefits of this sequence.

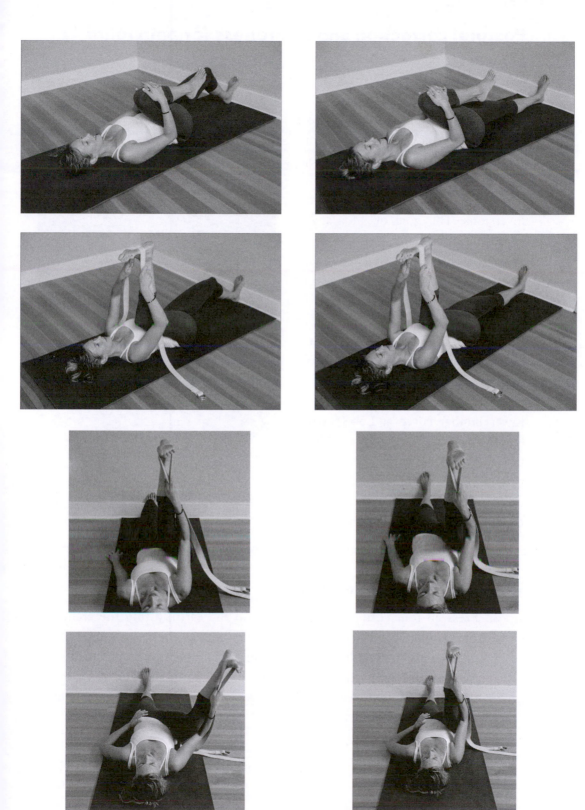

Figure 3.21 The Purna Yoga Low Back Series

Postural correction and awareness for pain relief

How to stand

Once your clients or students are able to stand upright, tell them to focus on practicing mountain pose (Tadasana). Standing correctly is one of the hardest poses in all of yoga but involves all of the foundational principles in standing postures and inversions. The goal of Tadasana is to maintain the normal curves of the spine so the muscles that have been working hard to "hold you up against gravity" can relax, as you find the optimal position where gravity can be absorbed by the skeleton and the muscles designed for postural control can be accessed and strengthened.

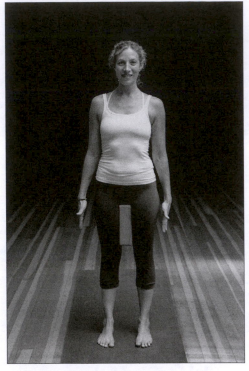

Figure 3.22 Mountain pose/Tadasana with proper alignment (with block between thighs)

The key is to maintain the lower lumbar curve at L5–S1 while lengthening the back of the body so that there is more space between each pair of vertebrae. This is called "axial extension," and occurs when you give the following instructions and your client or student follows them.

1. Place a block between the thighs, towards the pelvic floor, and stand with the feet hips' distance apart. This provides a stable base of support in line with the pelvis.

2. Press all four corners of your feet into the earth, lifting the arches. This proper contact with the ground energizes the leg muscles and prevents pronation (flat feet) and supination (outwardly arched feet) so that the hips and knees are in proper alignment. In addition, the more you ground into the earth, the more you will lengthen, so think about *rooting* in order to *lift*.

3. Engage your quadriceps by lifting the kneecaps up into the thighs. It is essential to fire the quadriceps in standing so that the legs hold the weight of the body, not the lower back, which is the more vulnerable part.

4. Squeeze the block with the inner thighs and try to push the block out the back. Relax the buttocks. This will create a subtle internal rotation action in the hip joint, which helps to relax the powerful gluteus maximus muscle and opens up the sacroiliac joint and lower back. Make sure that the knees stay pointing straight ahead, even though the thighs are rolling inward.

5. Maintaining the internal rotation, locate the lower belly (the area between the navel and the pubic bone) and lift the lower belly towards your head. This action is very important for maintaining length in the lower back as well as stabilizing the core. As you lift the pit of the abdomen (POA), you can feel the sacrum descending towards the earth. *Avoid tucking*, as this creates a posterior pelvic tilt—which puts excessive pressure on the discs and vertebrae, since the natural curve of the lower back is lost (see Figure 3.23 a.).

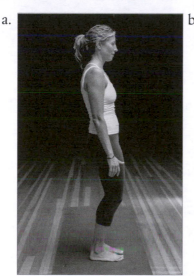 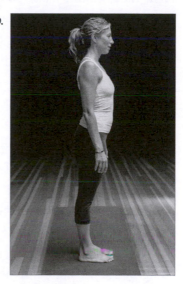

Figure 3.23 Posterior pelvic tilt: a. the result of "tucking" the tailbone vs. b. neutral spine

In addition, tucking occurs with a strong contraction of the buttocks, which creates more tension in the lower back and sacroiliac joint.

6. Move the shoulder blades away from the ears and lift the sternum. When you descend the shoulder blades, it helps to open the chest and relax the upper trapezius (neck) muscle.

7. Lengthen through the crown of the head. This creates length through the entire spine from the inside out, and prevents a forward head posture. Hold this properly aligned stance for one to two minutes. Release, and repeat two times every hour.

How to sit

Sitting will often be the most painful position for students or clients with back pain, as it increases the forces on the lower back. Many of my clients cannot sit for an extended period of time, and have a difficult time especially when sitting on airplanes for long flights. Showing your clients this technique will empower them to create less compression in the spine and allow for a comfortable seated position.

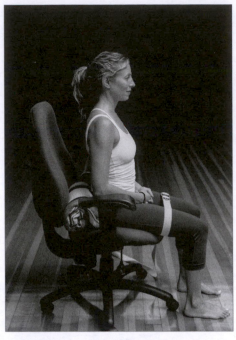

Figure 3.24 How to sit to reduce back pain

1. First, they should make sure that their hips are higher than the knees (best at a 30° angle) and their feet are planted on the floor.

2. Have them roll up a towel or sheet and place the roll behind the sacrum. Please note that the roll should not be placed in the lumbar spine, but at the very base of the spine behind the sacrum. This will help push the sacrum forward, allowing the lower back to maintain its natural lordotic curve.

3. Invite them to place a yoga belt around their thighs so that the thighs are hips' distance apart. This will help prevent the thighs from rolling out to the side, which can create more compression in the spine and compromise the natural lumbar curve.

4. Encourage them to be sure to get up and walk around every hour at minimum. Every half-hour would be preferable.

CASE STUDY: MARK

Treatment Session 1

Let us return to Mark, who is still in a lot of pain. He was able to stand and walk, but was shifted towards the left. He was unable to stand, walk, or sit for more than 10 to 15 minutes, but he had to return to work after taking a week off.

Upon further inquiry, Mark revealed that he was tired of his job and was eager to retire. He was holding on for another five years so that he would be vested in a retirement package that would support him and his wife. In addition, his wife, too, had chronic back pain and was not working, which made him feel more responsible for providing for them both. Mark felt trapped and in pain.

Over the last few years Mark had had bouts of back pain and had developed specific protective mechanisms to hold tension. He held a great deal of tension in his upper trapezius, and his back muscles were hard and tense from overuse. Essentially, his muscles were working overtime to protect his spine, which was not aligned correctly. He had lost the curve in his lumbar spine and contracted his buttocks to stand and walk, which caused a "tucking" of the pelvis into a posterior pelvic tilt. This, in turn, created tightness in the hamstrings, and the tightness was exacerbated because Mark sat for long periods of time at the computer. His shoulders were rounded forward, creating tightness in the pectoral muscles and anterior displacement of the heads of the humerus. He also complained of chronic neck pain and headaches he had suffered for the past 15 years. He managed his pain by taking Tylenol daily.

After our first contact, Mark and I created a home program that consisted of:

- a breathing exercise to help him calm down and focus on exhalation, supine over folded blankets for chest opening and smooth, even breathing (Figure 3.25). In this position he extended his exhalations and immediately experienced a calming effect

a.

b.

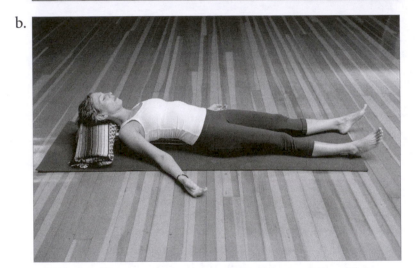

Figure 3.25 Supine chest opener for breathing and relaxation with two blankets
(folded accordion style): a. blanket position; b. full pose

- the low back series to decrease muscular tension
- traction (gentle) and positioning
- practice of correct standing and sitting postures, as illustrated above.

CHAPTER 4

Opening the Hips

The Key to Lower Back Health

There is a place inside all of us where everything is OK. Let's go there.

Aman Keays

Several years ago I experienced a trauma that revealed the body's power to respond to injury, threat, and challenge. I went with a friend to another friend's house to return an item that he had borrowed. The owner of the house was not home, and even though there was a dog inside, my friend assured me that if we entered the house quietly and let the owner's pet sniff me, all would be well. And so we went into the house. The dog came up to me, sniffed my hand, seemed to be at peace with my presence, and walked away slowly. My friend and I stayed in the house for a moment talking, when, with no warning, I felt a stinging, sharp pain in my right torso. The dog had sunk its teeth into my waist and was not letting go.

I let out a scream of shock more than of pain, and my friend came to my side to prise the dog off me. When he succeeded, I ran outside and closed the door behind me. Immediately, without any hesitation or thought, I dropped to my knees and folded in on myself, a position which is called child's pose (Ananda Balasana) in yoga. I stayed in that position, unable to move, for 15 or 20 minutes. My friend tried to get me to move, to get into the car and go, but I felt I would faint or die if I left the safety and comfort of that position.

Luckily the wounds were not deep and I recovered quickly, but I believe the shock of the event definitely left its mark.

In the days following that experience, and still, to this day, what remains with me is my instinctive response to the attack—to curl up into a ball and freeze once I was out of immediate danger. My body knew exactly what to do and was fully fired up to take charge of my survival. Although my intellect knew that I would be all right, my instincts and physical responses took control at that moment.

This experience illustrated to me how swiftly and intensely our bodies respond to fear and the need to protect ourselves. Our sympathetic nervous system kicks in immediately, short-circuiting the rational mind. The more I study the body and its rehabilitation, the more I see that the *physical body is a map of our mental and emotional state*. As David Berceli (2008) states in his book *The Evolutionary Trauma Release Process*, "The emotional pain we carry within us isn't just in our heads. It's also etched into our muscles" (p.37). This chapter will explore the hip-related muscles that can contribute to back pain, and also the hidden ways in which physical injury and emotional trauma can remain gripped in the body as chronic back pain. We will explore both physical exercises and emotional tools that together can inspire your students and clients with the courage to let go.

Back pain, trauma, and the psoas

One of the muscles that pulled me into that curled-up position on the floor is called the psoas major, a large muscle that functions to bring the trunk towards the hip or the hip towards the trunk. It is one of the main muscles that reacts in the "fight or flight" state, when we are in stress and need to run away, fight the enemy, or freeze—as most animals do, and as I did when danger threatened. The psoas is considered a powerful hip flexor, but its effect on the spine is just as important, for the two psoas muscles originate on each side of the vertebrae T12–L5. The psoas then joins the iliacus muscle and interconnects with the diaphragm above it to form a triad of muscles that respond to one another.

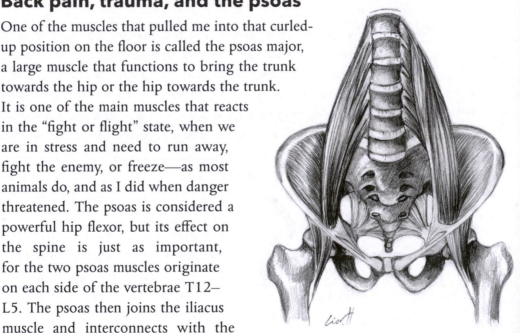

Figure 4.1 Psoas major and the iliacus muscle

Movement educator Liz Koch explores just this one muscle in *The Psoas Book* (1981/2012), for it is a fascinating and mysterious one that seems to behave in both voluntary and involuntary ways. In an online article on PilatesUnion.com, "Pulling it all together: Psoas, fear & core strength," Koch (2011) writes:

When fear strikes, responsiveness, not knee jerk reaction, saves lives. Responsiveness is the key to survival. Different from brute strength, core integrity is found quite literally at the center of our being. The muscle/tissue responsible for this inner power is called the Psoas (pronounced so-as). Located behind the abdominals, organs, and major artery, the Psoas literally grows out of the sides of the spine and spans from solar plexus to inner thigh, and it is the major player responsible for the fear response. Prime mover of our flee/fight/freeze survival instinct, it is your Psoas that drives you into that fast run, thrusts that high kick in the air, rolls your spine into a ball protecting you from a blow or the impact of falling through space, and in a heightened state of fear, stops you dead in your tracks. Only a supple, dynamic, and quite frankly expressive Psoas provides the resiliency, agility, and subtle balance necessary to achieve a sense of safety in a time of trauma. (Koch 1981/2012)

We need this fear response in order to survive, but what happens if we perceive that we are in a state of stress or trauma on a daily basis?

Our state of mind, and state of stress, can actually create a heightened fear response even when we are not in immediate danger. This cycle can keep us in chronic pain even when we should be in a relaxed state. We have seen this in the stories of Dan (who "manufactures tension") and Mark (whose physical injury was exacerbated by his sense of "feeling trapped").

The psoas is only one of the major muscles that act on both the spine and the hips. In order to understand how profound the impact of these muscles can be on spinal health and mobility, as well as back pain, we must examine all the muscles that surround the hip and pelvis. These muscles can be viewed as cables that control the mobility and flexibility of the pelvis as it adapts to the needs of the spine. The lower back is directly connected to the pelvis via the L5–S1 joint, and therefore every movement of the spine has a direct effect on the pelvis and sacrum—and vice versa. They cannot be viewed as separate from one another. The information below will allow you to help your students or clients discover this direct relationship between the pelvis, sacrum, and spine.

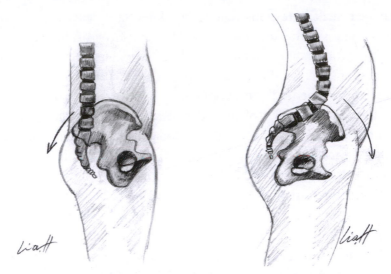

Figure 4.2 Relationship between the pelvis and spine during a posterior and anterior tilt

PRACTICE TIP 9
FEEL THE EFFECTS OF THE PELVIS ON THE SPINE

Sit on a cushion or yoga block with your legs crossed. Using your pelvis, start to shift your weight backwards and notice how the spine will begin to round. Then tip your pelvis forward and notice how this encourages a greater lumbar curve. Continue weight shifting in many different directions and notice how each subtle movement affects your spine and the surrounding musculature. Even the slightest tilt of the pelvis anteriorly or posteriorly has a profound effect on the lower back.

How hip muscles affect your spine

1. Iliopsoas and rectus femoris (hip flexors)

The iliopsoas muscle is made up of two muscles, the psoas major and the iliacus. In the abdominal area they are two distinct muscles, but become one muscle, the iliopsoas, as they join together at the level of the pelvis and anterior thigh. The psoas major originates on the lateral surfaces of the vertebral bodies and discs of T12 and L1–L5. The iliacus originates in the iliac fossa of the pelvis. They join together to cross the hip joint and insert on the lesser trochanter of the femur (see Figure 4.3).

The rectus femoris is one of four muscles that make up the quadriceps and is the only part of the quads that crosses over the hip joint. It originates on the anterior inferior iliac spine of the pelvis, as well as from a groove above the rim of the acetabulum, and joins the other three muscles of the quadriceps (vastus lateralis, vastus medialis and vastus intermedius) to insert into a common tendon on the patella (see Figure 4.4).

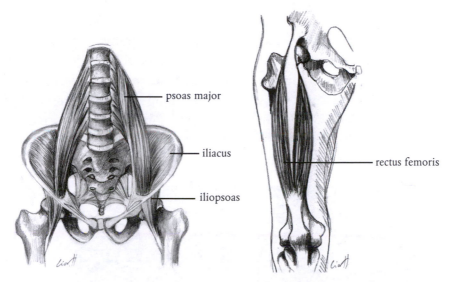

*Figure 4.3 Iliopsoas muscle
(psoas major and iliacus)*

Figure 4.4 Rectus femoris muscle

Both of these muscles act as hip flexors and, when tight or restricted, pull the pelvis into an anterior tilt. When the pelvis is fixed in an anteriorly tilted position, the lower back is forced to overarch in order to compensate. This tends to create an exaggerated curve in the lumbar spine, which, in turn, causes compression in the lower back (see Figure 4.5).

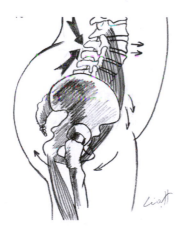

Figure 4.5 How the iliopsoas and rectus femoris muscles pull the pelvis into an anterior tilt

Once these muscles are stretched out, the pelvis can settle back into its natural position and the natural lumbar curve can be restored. But until those muscles are lengthened, your students may experience compression in their lumbar spine during poses that require supple and long hip flexors.

The most common yoga postures that can create compression for those with tight hip flexors include Virabhadrasana I/warrior I (see Figure 4.6) and most back bends, such as Ustrasana/camel and Urdhva Dhanurasana/Wheel. It is important for teachers and therapists to be able to identify when a student is hinging in their lower back in these poses instead of *lengthening* as they extend the lumbar spine. Most often, stretching both the iliopsoas and rectus femoris muscles can alleviate the pain and compression these students may experience in the posture. We will be exploring multiple techniques to accomplish this later in this chapter.

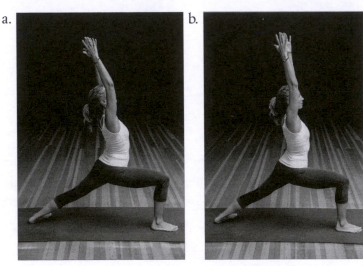

Figure 4.6 Virabhadrasana I/warrior I:
a. with overarching in the lower back due to tightness in the hip flexors;
b. with length in lumbar spine

2. The hamstrings (hip extensors and knee flexors)

The hamstrings are the muscles of the posterior thigh: semitendinosus, semimembranosus, and biceps femoris (long and short head). These muscles make up the bulk of the back of the thigh and create the space behind the knee with their tendons as borders. Three of the four hamstrings cross over both the hip and knee joints and are responsible for hip extension and knee flexion. One of the hamstrings (the short head of the biceps femoris) crosses over the knee joint and is responsible only for knee flexion.

The semitendinosus, semimembranosus, and long head of biceps femoris muscles all originate on the ischial tuberosities of the pelvis, also known as the "sitting bones" in the yoga world. The short head of the biceps is the only member of the hamstring family that originates on the posterior femur, and therefore has no role in hip extension (it only affects knee flexion). The semitendinosus attaches on the medial surface of the tibia, while the semimembranosus

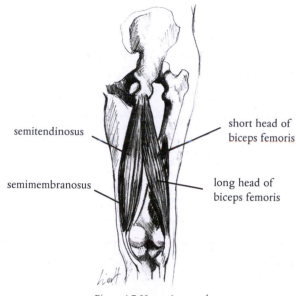

semitendinosus

semimembranosus

short head of
biceps femoris

long head of
biceps femoris

Figure 4.7 Hamstring muscles

attaches to the medial condyle of the tibia. The biceps femoris (both long and short head) attaches onto the lateral head of the fibula.

Because of the hamstrings' attachment to the sitting bones (ischial tuberosities), decreased flexibility in the hamstrings results in an increased posterior pelvic tilt. This backward tilt of the pelvis results in a decreased lumbar curve and the tendency to push the pelvis forward, the result being a shortened lower back with a tendency to "sit on" the ligaments of the spine and pelvis. This flattening of the lumbar curve also increases the amount of pressure on the lower lumbar vertebrae, as it is not bearing the weight of the body at the appropriate and ideal angle for which it was designed.

Stretching the hamstrings frees up the pelvis so it can move back to its natural state and maintain a natural lumbar curve.

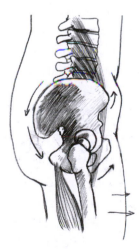

Figure 4.8 How tight hamstrings create a posterior pelvic tilt

3. Piriformis (hip external rotator)

The piriformis muscle runs from the anterior surface of the sacrum to the outer hip and is a powerful external hip rotator (see Figure 4.9). When this muscle is tight or inflamed it pulls your hips into external rotation, which results in the feet turning out to the sides, combined with the tendency to push the pelvis forward, thereby compressing the sacroiliac joint and shortening the lumbar spine.

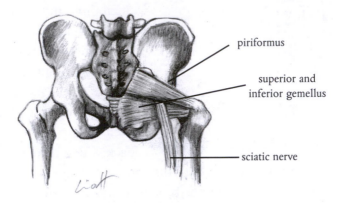

Figure 4.9 The piriformis muscle

In addition, this muscle runs directly over the sciatic nerve, and when tight or inflamed can create symptoms that are similar to sciatica. This condition is called "piriformis syndrome" and relates to pain and tingling in the buttock and down the posterior thigh and leg, along the pathway of the sciatic nerve. It can be due to strain or overuse, as well as anatomical differences that create compression of the nerve behind or within the muscle belly.

When the external rotators are lengthened, the feet can return to a neutral position and compression on the lower back is decreased.

4. Gluteus medius, gluteus minimus and tensor fasciae latae (hip abductors)

The hip abductors include three main muscles that all originate on the lateral aspect of the ilium (part of the pelvis). These muscles are the gluteus medius, gluteus minimus, and tensor fasciae latae. The two gluteal muscles attach to the greater trochanter of the femur, while the tensor fasciae latae inserts in the iliotibial band on the lateral aspect of the thigh.

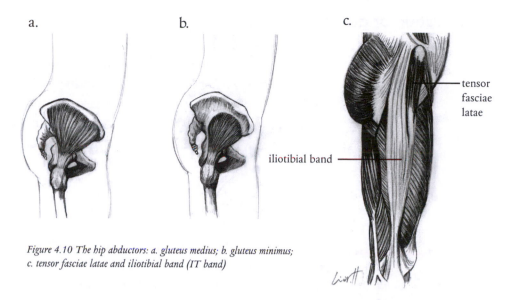

a.　b.　c.

tensor
fasciae
latae

iliotibial band

Figure 4.10 The hip abductors: a. gluteus medius; b. gluteus minimus;
c. tensor fasciae latae and iliotibial band (IT band)

These muscles become tight from almost every activity other than yoga. Most sports, including cycling, running, hiking, swimming, and surfing, tend to build strength in the hip abductors, but also create tightness in this area, especially in the iliotibial band. Sedentary individuals also tend to be tight in these muscles, but for different reasons. Individuals who spend a lot of time sitting in a chair will find their outer hips to be tight and their inner thighs (hip adductors) to be weak, as their legs tend to roll out to the sides while seated. In addition, sedentary individuals tend to adopt a standing position with their feet turned out, as it provides a greater base of support and requires little core activation. For all these reasons, there is less internal rotation available in the hip joint, tightness in the hip abductors, and weakness in the hip adductors, pelvic floor, and abdominals. This common triad of dysfunction creates the "perfect storm" for an episode of lower back pain and increased compression in the spine.

Opening up the outer hips and hip abductors will free up the hip so that internal rotation is available to your students. They can begin to strengthen their internal rotators of the hip and adductors in addition to their core. Flexible outer hip muscles lead to more space in the lower back and easier access to the muscles required for correct postural stability.

5. The adductor group (hip adductors)

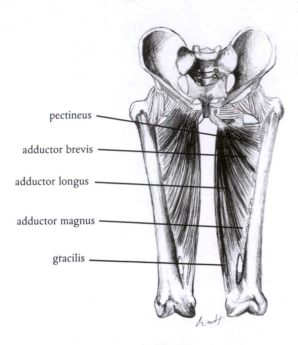

pectineus

adductor brevis

adductor longus

adductor magnus

gracilis

Figure 4.11 The adductor group

In the context of our discussion, the muscles of the adductor group tend to be weak in individuals with lower back pain. Because the tendency of the body is to be tight and stronger in external rotation, these muscles are often forgotten and remain under-utilized. The adductor group is also part of the "core" of the body, and therefore a strong and supple adductor group will encourage strength in the pelvic floor and deep abdominal muscles.

The adductor group is made up of the following muscles: adductor brevis, adductor longus, adductor magnus, adductor minimus, pectineus, gracilis, and obturator externus. They all originate on different areas on the pubis and ischium and insert into the medial aspect of the femur bone.

Putting it all together

The interrelationships among these main hip muscles highlight one of the limitations of conventional medical management of back pain—its tendency to look at and treat only the specific area where there is pain or obvious injury as seen on a radiograph or MRI. When we approach the body this way, we treat the symptoms of back pain with medication, local injections, anesthetics, and surgery, which aims to correct or remove the problem. The trouble with this approach is that it does not address the *reason* for the pain, making it likely that the pain will return in either the same place or an adjacent area in the future.

Consider this example: After swimming in the ocean one day, I notice a dull pain in my shoulder that worsens when I try to lift my arm overhead. I ignore these symptoms and continue swimming until one day I find myself in excruciating pain and cannot continue to use my shoulder at all. At this point

I go to my doctor, who prescribes anti-inflammatories and suspects a rotator cuff (supraspinatus) tear or tendonitis. He tells me to rest my shoulder and to consider surgery if the pain does not subside.

Yet no one has inquired about the form of my swimming stroke. Had I been evaluated from a more holistic point of view, it would have been obvious that my shoulders were curved forward with an increased rounding (kyphosis) in my upper back.

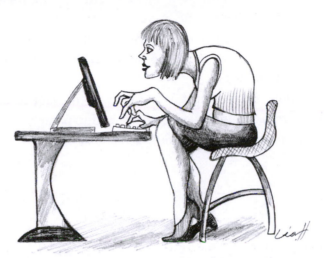

Figure 4.12 Posture contributing to shoulder impingement in swimmers.
Pain and dysfunction will reoccur until this posture is corrected

In this position, every time I lift my arm overhead during my swimming stroke, I compress the tendons of the long head of the biceps as well as the supraspinatus tendon (which is part of the rotator cuff). Even if I begin to feel better with rest and medication, the source of the problem has not been identified, and the minute I begin to swim consistently again, the same problem will emerge because its source is my poor technique. The only way to heal the shoulder and remain pain-free is to correct the faulty posture, which continues to compress the tendons in my shoulder joint. I would need to stretch my anterior chest musculature and strengthen my upper back muscles in order to correctly align my shoulder joint and free it from compression.

The same process happens inside your body in a more subtle way when you feel back pain. When your muscles around the pelvis and spine are tight, unnecessary pressure is transmitted to the lower back, which inevitably breaks down in some way depending on the imbalance. If you can free up these muscles so that the pressure is diminished, you will be free from pain.

Back to basic concepts

Because of its direct effect on the pelvis and lumbar spine, *tightness in the hip musculature is one of the most common causes of lower back pain.* This brings us back to the concept of *peeling the onion* discussed in Chapter 1. While the pain or inflammation may be in the lower back, once the initial phase calms down, we can begin to peel down to the root of the problem. The swimming analogy shows us that when the tight muscles in the hip are stretched out and weak muscles are strengthened, the pressure is diminished and the spine can be free to heal without further recurrence. Opening the hips enables us to *maintain the natural curves of the spine,* another of the basic principles necessary for complete healing to occur.

In order to work on the hips, we need to open them in every possible direction. There are six main movements in the hips, namely *flexion, extension, abduction, adduction, external rotation,* and *internal rotation.*

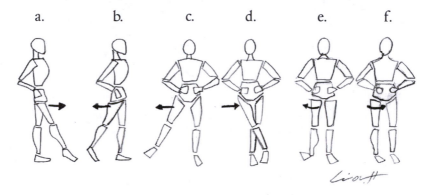

Figure 4.13 Movements available in the hip joint: a. flexion; b. extension; c. abduction; d. adduction; e. external rotation; f. internal rotation

In addition, there are also two subtle movements that are related to the hip joint. These are *traction* and *contraction.* Traction refers to moving the joint surfaces away from one another, while contraction (or compression) refers to moving the joint surfaces towards one another, thereby decreasing the space in the joint.

When dealing with joints that are stable, such as the hip joint with its strong muscles and ligaments, it is important to create more *traction* in that joint, meaning more space and more flexibility. But for joints that by nature lack stability, such as the shoulder joint, which can easily dislocate, we focus on *contraction,* or keeping the shoulder in joint during many yoga postures, especially when bearing our own weight with the arms. To return to our basic principles, we always must *balance stability with mobility.*

The Purna Yoga Hip Opening Series designed by Aadil Palkhivala is a wonderfully effective sequence that includes moving the hips in all six directions, *along with traction*. When done with awareness to the subtle instructions, this series can help free up your students' or clients' hips and pelvises, thereby decreasing compression in the spine. I have personally seen many of my clients transform their bodies and free themselves from lower back pain after simply doing this one sequence. It's that powerful!

The Purna Yoga Hip Opening Series: Six directions of movement with traction

Your clients or students will need a strap for this exercise. It can be done with the bottom foot against a wall, which facilitates a greater contraction in the bottom leg, or in the middle of the room. The instructions are stated here, as you should give them to the student or client.

1. Supta Padangusthasana

Hip flexion—stretches the hamstrings

- Place a strap around the right foot just above the heel at the bottom of the arch. Keep the left knee bent and the left foot on the floor. Slowly straighten the right leg.

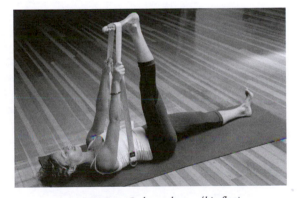

Figure 4.14 Supta Padangusthasana / hip flexion

- *It is important that you only raise your right leg as high as you can while maintaining an extended knee. The height of your leg does not matter*—what matters is that you energize your thigh muscles and keep the knee straight so that the hamstrings can effectively stretch without strain. If your knee is bending, move the leg away from your head until you can straighten the knee and contract the front thigh muscles (the quadriceps). This action will create a relaxation response in the hamstrings (a concept called reciprocal inhibition) and will encourage your hamstrings to open naturally.

- Slowly straighten your left leg as much as possible, pressing the left heel away from you (or into the wall) as you lift your lower belly toward your head.

- Roll the left inner thigh down towards the floor, keeping the left knee and toes pointed upward—in other words, do not let the foot roll out to the side.

- Engage the quadriceps as you move the right outer hip away from your head, keeping the frontal hip bones level while creating space in your right hip joint.

- Keep the arms straight and press the shoulder blades into the floor so that the chest stays open.

- Hold for nine deep breaths, and then switch sides.

2. Parivrtta Supta Padangusthasana

Hip adduction—stretches the piriformis muscle, the tensor fasciae latae (TFL), and the iliotibial (IT) band

- Set up as in 1 above.

- Place the strap around the right outer ankle and heel and hold the strap in your left hand from the inside. Then place the "L" of the index finger and thumb of the right hand into your right hip crease.

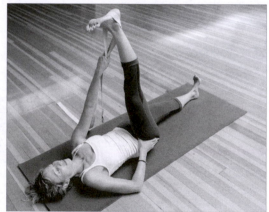

- With the right hand in the right hip crease, breathe in, and on the exhalation push your hip away from your head, creating more traction in the hip joint.

Figure 4.15 Parivrtta Supta Padangusthasana/hip adduction

- Extend through both inner heels.

- Gently take your right leg towards the left, keeping your foot in line with your left shoulder. *Do not let the foot pass the opposite shoulder; if you do you will overshoot the muscles we are aiming to stretch.*

- Lift the lower belly as you traction the right hip away from the head. Traction is accomplished by pressing the right hand into the right groin and moving the femur bone away from the head.

- Hold for nine breaths, and then switch sides.

3. Parsva Supta Padangusthasana

Hip abduction—stretches the hip adductors

- Set up as in 1 above, wedging a folded blanket under the edge of the right buttock. (This will help support the outer hip and keep the pelvis from tipping over to the right side.)

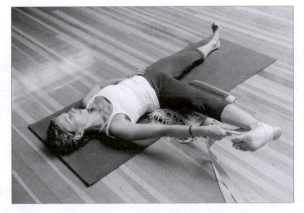

Figure 4.16 Parsva Supta Padangusthasana / hip abduction

- Place the belt around the right inner ankle and heel and hold it with the right hand from the outside. Then place your left hand on top of your left hip to keep it moving towards the left.

- Press through both heels and lift the lower belly.

- Take your right leg out to the right side, leading with the heel.

- Keep the outer edge of your right foot parallel with the floor. The tendency in this pose is for the foot to turn outward towards the floor. Instead, keep the heel in line with the pinky toe at all times.

- Maintain traction in the hip by contracting the quadriceps in the top leg and moving the femur bone away from the head.

- Hold for nine breaths, and then switch sides.

4. Duryodhansana

Internal hip rotation—increases internal rotation in the hip joint and stretches the psoas muscle

a.

b.

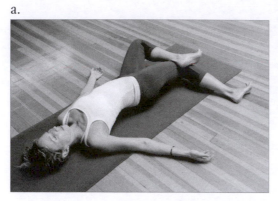 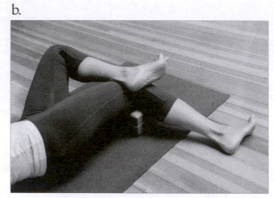

Figure 4.17 a. Internal rotation; b. internal rotation with block support under knee

- Lie on your back with your feet on the floor and knees bent at a 90° angle.

- Step your right foot out to the right one shin length. Flex both feet, and then bring the right knee down towards the left ankle. Then place the left ankle over the right thigh.

- Let the right buttock come off the ground in this pose, but make sure to lift the lower belly in order to maintain the integrity of the lumbar spine.

Important! If there is any pain in the right knee, place a block or blanket underneath for support.

- If there is no pain in your right knee joint, begin to move the knee away from the head so the focus is on creating traction in the hip while in internal rotation. Do not press the knee towards the floor—emphasize length instead, but let it drop downwards on its own.

- Lengthen your thighbone away from your head as you pull the lower belly toward your head.

- Hold for nine breaths, and then switch sides.

5. Supta Janu Padasthilasana

External hip rotation—increases external rotation in the hip joint

a.

b.

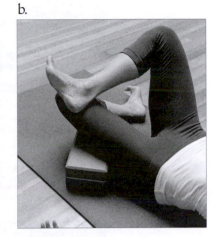

Figure 4.18 a. External rotation; b. with block for support

- Lie on your back with your feet on the floor, hips' width apart, and your knees bent at a 90° angle.

- Slide the left ankle behind the right foot and then place your right ankle on top of the left knee, opening both knees out to the sides. Place a block or blanket under your left thigh in order to keep the pelvis level.

- Make sure your torso is lined up with the yoga mat.

- Lift the lower belly as you traction both hips away from your head.

- Hold for nine breaths, and then switch sides.

6. Eka Pada Supta Virasana

Increases hip extension and stretches the quadriceps and hip flexors

a.

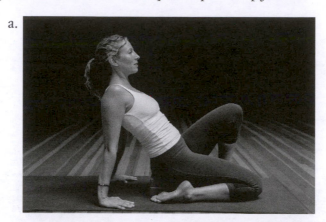

b.

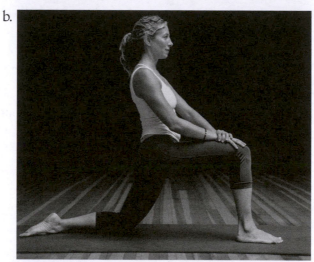

c.

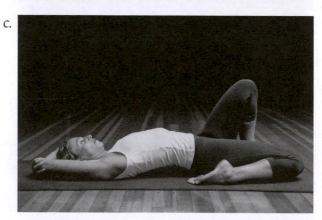

Figure 4.19 Eka Pada Supta Virasana/hip extension: a. modified with block under buttocks; b. option to modify if there is knee pain; c. final position

- Begin on your hands and knees. Bring your knees together and your heels out wider than your hips to sit into Virasana on a yoga block.

- Bring your left foot forward and place the sole of your foot onto the floor.

- *Important! Make sure the right knee is on the floor and that there is no pain in the knees.* If this position is uncomfortable, place another block under the buttocks. If this is still painful, come out of this pose and work on a lunge as a modification (see Figure 4.19 b.). There should *never* be pain in the knees in this position.

- Keep your right knee in line with your right hip. Place your hands behind you and push down to lift your hips. Extend the tailbone forward so that you feel a greater stretch in the front thigh of the bottom leg. Place your right sitting bone back onto the block and press your right inner knee to the floor as you lift your lower belly.

- If you are comfortable here, and the right knee does not lift off the ground, you can remove the block and rest on your elbows or lie all the way onto your back.

- Hold for nine breaths, and then switch sides.

PRACTICE TIP 10

USING THE HIP OPENING SERIES AS A DIAGNOSTIC TOOL

As you go through the hip opening series, begin to pay attention to any asymmetries that may present themselves. You should pay attention to two things:

1. Is there one movement that is more restricted in one direction than the other? (For example, you have more mobility in external rotation, but internal rotation is challenging for you.)

2. Is there one side that is tighter than the other during the same movement? (For example, your right leg can go up to 90° in hip flexion, but your left feels tight at 75°.)

Pay close attention to these imbalances, as they will give you a picture of where you need to work in order to realign.

Once you identify one movement or one side that is more restricted than the other, you can work more on that side in order to create more symmetry. For example: You should do Exercise 1 (hip flexion) on the left leg twice as much as on the right, if the left side is limited. You can begin on the left, stretch the right, and then return to the left side for another repetition. This will create more balance in your body.

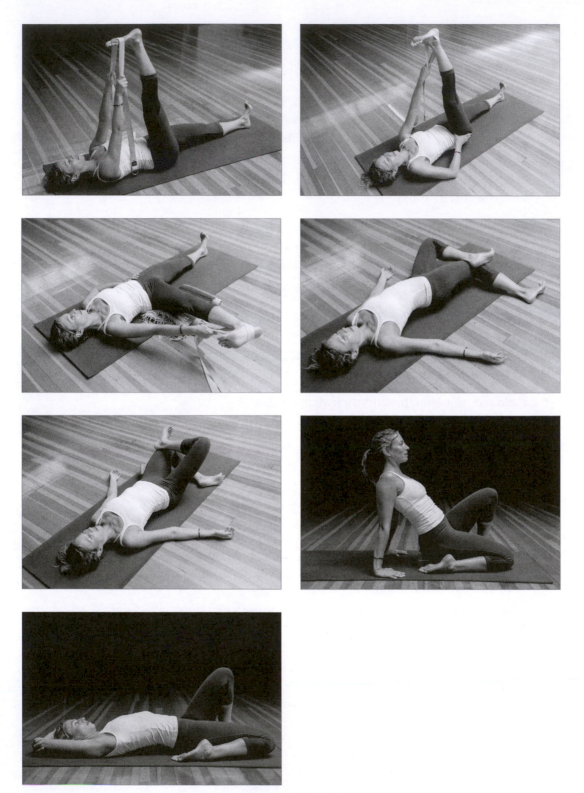

Figure 4.20 The Purna Yoga Hip Opening Series

Hip strengthening exercises

In addition to opening the hips, you will need to continuously *balance mobility with stability* by strengthening the weak muscles of the pelvis that contribute to poor posture and faulty movement patterns. The muscles that tend to be weak are mainly the adductors and internal rotators of the hip—as well as the pelvic floor musculature. The beauty of yoga is that it does not allow us to do what our body wants to do "naturally" but encourages the recruitment of smaller, postural muscles that help maintain health in the spine.

For example, when sitting with legs extended, the tendency is for the toes to fall out to the sides, favoring external rotation in the hips. In this pose, the

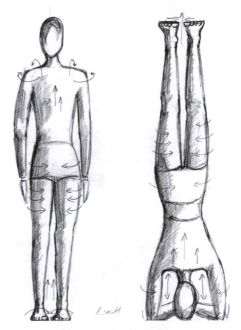

Figure 4.21 Leg action in Tadasana/mountain pose and Sirsasana/headstand

instruction is just the opposite and is very challenging to accomplish correctly. We are encouraged to create internal rotation in the hips by drawing the inner thighs towards the floor; activate the pelvic floor and adductors by squeezing the legs together; and make the inner legs longer by pushing through the big toe mound, while pulling the pinky toe back towards the hip joint.

These instructions are found over and over again in descriptions of poses, both standing and inverted, in which the legs are together, the two most apparent being Tadasana/mountain pose and Sirsasana/headstand. It is probably more apparent in headstand, as the "aliveness" of the legs is crucial in maintaining the balance and decreasing weight on the neck and spine.

In each of these poses the instructions are to "wake up" the inner thighs by pressing out through the inner heels. A slight action of internal rotation in the inner thighs keeps the knees pointing straight ahead, which in turn helps prevent the feet from rolling out to the sides. In addition, there is a sense of squeezing the inner thighs towards one another, which strengthens the hip adductors (inner thigh muscles) and pelvic floor.

Below are some of my favorite poses to build strength and stability in the hips and pelvis; again, the instructions are as you should give them to your students or clients.

1. Dandasana with strap above the ankles

- Sit on a blanket with your legs extended in front of you.

- *Make sure the sacrum is at a 90° angle to the floor by placing your hand on the area* (see Figure 4.22). If your sacrum is tilting backwards, place more height under your buttocks until it is perpendicular to the floor.

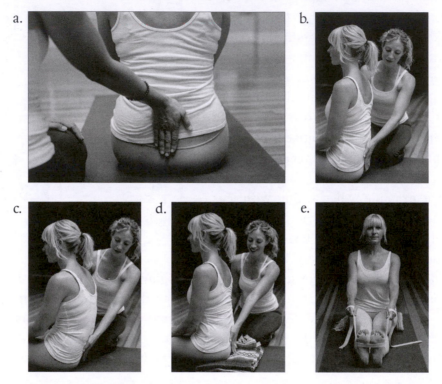

Figure 4.22 a. Placement of the hand on the sacrum; b. at 90° correctly; c. at less than 90°; d. elevated sitting to achieve proper positioning in the spine in Dandasana; e. Dandasana with straps around toe mounds

- Place a strap around the arches of your feet just above the heels, and hold the strap with both hands.

- Press the inner heels forward as you press your thigh bones down towards the ground.

- Pull on the strap and lift your chest, moving the sacrum into your body.

- Squeeze your inner thighs towards one another, rolling the skin of the inner thighs down towards the ground.

- Keep your neck and shoulders relaxed, with the shoulder blades moving away from the ears. Work your legs hard in the pose, but find some relaxation in the neck and shoulders at the same time.

- Hold for nine breaths and relax. Repeat three times.

2. Tadasana with block between the legs

- Stand with your feet firmly planted on the ground, outer edges of the feet in line with the mat.

- Place a block lengthwise between your upper thighs.

- Squeeze the block between the thighs as you gently roll the inner thighs back. You should feel as if you are pushing the block backwards.

- Engage the quadriceps and feel the kneecaps lift up into the thigh muscles.

- Lift the lower belly and lengthen the lower back.

- Hold for nine breaths. Repeat three times.

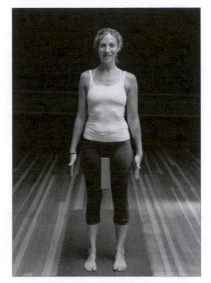

Figure 4.23 Tadasana with block

3. Wall squat with block between the legs

- Sit with your back and pelvis against the wall.

- Place the block between your upper thighs as you slowly bend your knees and come into a squat. *Caution: Never bring the buttocks lower than the hips, as it can hurt your knees.*

- Keeping the spine in line with the wall, hold here in a squatting position as you actively squeeze the block between your legs.

- Hold for 30 seconds to one minute. Repeat three times.

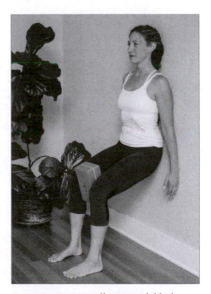

Figure 4.24 Wall squat with block

Poses that involve standing on one leg are also very helpful for strengthening an important muscle that affects gait and posture: the gluteus medius muscle. One such posture that is easy to practice is Vrksasana/tree pose, standing against the wall.

4. Vrksasana—standing against the wall

- Start by standing a few inches away from the wall, with your back towards the wall.

- Make sure your left foot is facing forward, and root down through all four corners of the foot of the standing leg.

- Engage the quadriceps by lifting the kneecap on the left leg.

- Turn the toes out on the right leg and place the right foot as high as possible into the left inner thigh/groin area. *Do not place the foot on the knee joint.* If your foot does not reach the groin area, place it above or below the knee joint. If balance is an issue, place your heel on the ankle, with the toes on the floor.

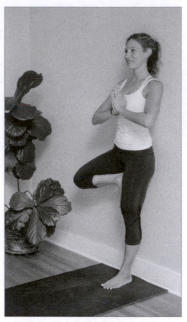

Figure 4.25 Vrksasana/tree pose

- Keep the pelvis level and open the right thigh out towards the wall. Focus on the external rotation coming from the hip joint, instead of pressing the knee back.

- Lift the pit of the abdomen.

- Avoid collapsing in the left hip by engaging the outer left thigh muscle, so that the pelvis remains level throughout the posture. (If your student collapses in the left outer hip, it is a sign of weakness in the gluteus medius muscle on the standing leg.)

All of the above exercises will help your students or clients open the hips and strengthen them in order to create the ideal alignment and prevent compression in their lower backs. However, it is important to come back to the emotional causes of tension as well, and address those in order to experience complete healing. Doing exercises without this inner awareness is just going through the motions without getting to the source. For the exercises to be truly effective we must face any emotional sources of our distress, the gripping which usually signals *fear and control.*

The emotional component: My story

When my mother was pregnant with me, my older sister Riva Leah, who was 18 months old at the time, was diagnosed with Tay Sachs disease. Tay Sachs is a genetic autoimmune disorder that affects many Ashkenazi Jews (Jews of Eastern European descent). At that time couples were not tested before they married, as they are now, for the disease is fatal in young children. Babies born with Tay Sachs appear completely healthy and develop as a normal child does; however, after a year or so, they begin to deteriorate slowly until eventually they lose muscle function and the ability to breathe. What makes this especially traumatic for new parents is that they have the time to bond with their seemingly healthy child, only to learn a year later that this child will slowly lose the ability to move and will eventually die. I can only imagine that pain and the constant reminder of loss as the child slowly begins to regress in front of their eyes over a long period of time. Most children die by the age of three.

When my parents received my sister's diagnosis, I was in my mother's womb. During my mother's pregnancy, my sister's health began to decline. I do not know for certain the extent of the grief my mother experienced at the time, but I do know that some of her pain and sorrow was passed on to me in the womb. When I was born, my sister was already quite disabled and could not sit up on her own; I saw this for myself in photos I found in an album hidden in the family basement. What I do know is that I was born while another child was dying. I was told that my grandmother came to help out, and I imagine that during my early days in this world I spent more time with her than with my parents. I believe that I experienced a deep feeling of abandonment and rejection, for my mother and father were not physically or emotionally available to me as a newborn and young child. When I was 18 months old, Riva Leah died.

My parents went on to have five more children and I became the oldest of the group. No one spoke of Riva Leah as we grew up. We children found a few black-and-white photos of Riva Leah as a baby in my mother's night table. She had dark eyes and dark hair and a beautiful smile; this was before she became ill. But for as long as I can remember, her name was never mentioned in the house. Life went on "as usual." My mother occupied herself with caring for the family and running the household; my father found his peace in silence, introversion, and social isolation. I believe that they never grieved together, and this created a wedge between them that deepened with the years until there was nothing left to hold them together.

So I grew up as a part of an intact middle-class family in suburban Montreal, a family that was fractured at its core. Both my parents were physically present but completely absent emotionally, for each of us as well as for each other.

Only later in life, after years of psychotherapy, yoga, and meditation, did I come to realize the devastating effect this history had on me and how far-reaching the effects were on my life and future relationships. When any child, especially a very young child, does not receive the love and safety he or she needs to develop a strong sense of self in relationship to the world, the nervous system develops in such a way that it is geared for survival. This causes important life choices to come from a place of fear. Without the *unconditional* love, support, and nurturing of a parent, children need to control their environment to create a sense of safety. But that security may depend on outside circumstances—friendships, physical appearance, possessions, accomplishments, romantic relationships, and career, among others. When the puzzle pieces fit together, such a person finds relief from the anxiety and uneasiness of his or her inner fragility. However, when things begin to unravel in life, even greater anxiety and stress return, and they are followed by a huge effort to get things back in balance one way or another.

This "survival" instinct, which results in a lack of trust in life and an inability to believe that we are supported, creates inner tension in those very muscles that contract during our fight or flight response. The body cannot distinguish its own stress level. Whether a tiger is chasing us, or we feel hopeless about healing an injury, or we feel insecure in our job, the sympathetic nervous system turns on, which in turn affects the muscles that contribute to our survival response. If we remain in this constant state of stress, a cycle of chronic tension and pain will be activated. A massage may make us feel better, but the body contracts again moments after getting home.

In order to experience true release, we need to find our way back to a parasympathetic state in which our muscles can relax and our bodies can function harmoniously. The only way to do this is to recognize the deep messages of fear and control that we carry in our body. If we continue to "suck it up" or "stuff it down," the tension will persist. Seeing this reality is difficult, as it puts us in a vulnerable state, for we may be forced to feel emotions we have suppressed for a long time: anger, hurt, sadness, disappointment, loneliness. Feeling fully is painful and uncomfortable. But if we do not recognize these deep feelings, we will not let go and allow ourselves to heal. We have to walk through the darkness to get to the light at the end of the tunnel—or, in yogic terms, we must take root in the mud before growing into the lotus flower of enlightenment.

The following practice tip, adapted from Koch, may help your students or clients to discover long-suppressed feelings, and by observing those, let them go. Deep, true relaxation may follow.

PRACTICE TIP 11

CONSTRUCTIVE RELAXATION POSE (CRP)

Be honest with yourself. Start to notice where in your life you are gripping and holding on for control. Where do you go to for comfort from the reality that we are really not in control of our lives? Food, work, relationships, sex, drugs, alcohol, shopping, exercise—yes, exercise can be a way of escape.

- Lie on your back with your knees bent and allow the feelings to surface. Begin to allow any uncomfortable feeling to arise and try not to run away from it. Stay with it. Notice how this affects your breath and your body.

- Now, place your hands on your frontal hipbones and allow the knees to touch.

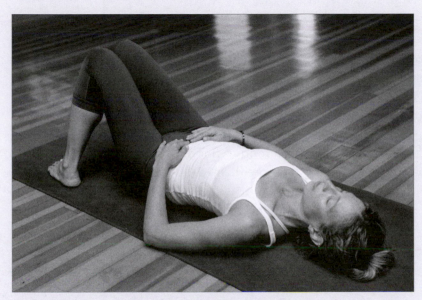

Figure 4.26 Constructive relaxation pose

- Inhale, and observe your belly rising into your hands. Exhale, and release any tension in your body. Feel your lower back spread wide open onto the earth; feel your tailbone extending away from your head. Feel your hip creases and groin soften and relax deep into the body.

- Hold this position for 10–15 minutes.

It may be difficult to stay still for so long. You may find your mind racing or your body hurting. Stay with it. Allow these feelings to surface and move through you. Allow yourself to truly relax, for once.

We cannot experience this type of awareness if we are moving all the time. It is necessary to *slow down* and *pay attention*. Purna Yoga helps us with this process, but we must find time to be still in order to hear what our body is telling us. This takes a great deal of courage and patience. But these kinds of self-study and meditative practice techniques are tools that will serve you for the rest of your life, long past the time you have opened your hips and healed your back. We will explore additional techniques to help with this process of self-exploration in Chapter 8, "Getting to the Heart of the Matter: Looking Inward."

CASE STUDY: MARK

Treatment Session 2

Mark has been doing his exercises daily. He feels more at ease and less stressed about the future, but is beginning to notice how tight he is and how he contracts all his big muscles at the same time. He has begun to experience a new awareness of how tight his hips really are. He wants to relax his back muscles but does not seem to know how.

Mark is no longer shifted to the left, and he is tolerating standing and sitting for longer periods of time. He still has difficulty while sitting for more than 20–30 minutes at a computer, and he still experiences pain when bending forward, although it is less intense than it was on initial evaluation.

Mark and I have talked about his fear of the future. He admits that he stays in his job out of fear that he will not be provided for by receiving a good enough retirement package if he leaves too early. He notices an increase in his pain on Sunday evenings, when he anticipates returning to his job. He realizes that he may even have gone into engineering initially out of pressure from his family to have a "good, solid profession" and has ignored many of the activities that gave him joy as a young adult. He misses playing basketball and painting, both of which he cannot do because of his chronic back pain.

After Session 2, Mark leaves with a few new exercises to add to his home program, which include:

- the Purna Yoga Hip Opening Series—to help free up his pelvis and spine
- Tadasana with a block between his legs—with the emphasis on building strength in his weaker hip muscles and keeping his shoulders and neck relaxed (i.e. turning off the muscles he usually contracts when stressed)

- wall squat with block (as above)
- constructive relaxation pose—with an emphasis on letting go of physical holding patterns. We also added a mantra to this exercise at the beginning: "I trust that I will have all I need in life. I am safe and supported."

CHAPTER 5

Demystifying the Sacroiliac Joint

I hope your sacrum finds its home.

A fellow student at Full Circle Yoga

I met Anna while she was enrolled in a yoga teacher training program. The more I came to know and understand her, the more her journey toward healing resembled my own. During the training she struggled to participate in many of the classes, due to chronic back pain. She was uncertain about continuing the training and was feeling discouraged and depressed by her longstanding physical limitations. The curious thing about Anna's pain was that it seemed to center on her sacroiliac joints—the joints that connect the sacrum to the uppermost bones of the pelvis on either side. Yet her pain didn't follow any specific pattern.

Anna's back pain began when she was a child. An avid athlete and gymnast, she would wear a back brace and was told to "work through the pain." Anna experienced periods where she was pain-free, but even as a young adult she felt debilitating pain in her lower back that caused her to miss several weeks of classes while she was in college.

At age 27 Anna moved to San Diego with her husband and began practicing Vinyasa and Power Yoga in addition to participating in triathlons and long-distance running. It was then that she felt a sharp pain in her back that caused her to stop all her activities. This time, the pain did not go away.

Anna was determined to find a solution to the chronic pain that kept her from doing the activities she loved most. She turned to traditional physical therapy, sports medicine doctors, and chiropractors for help. But even though she would feel some temporary relief, her pain would return with a vengeance. She felt she needed to find an alternative, outside of the western medical model, because that approach was just not working. In addition to the pain returning, she felt that she wasn't being heard or understood when she described her baffling condition.

When we began to work together privately, it became apparent that her sacroiliac joint would go out in different directions each week. There seemed to be neither rhyme nor reason for the dysfunction. Eventually she was able to identify one thing that made the pain worse—long periods of emotional stress. Soon we realized that she was using the wrong muscles—namely the bigger muscle groups—to create pelvic stability, rather than using more subtle internal, postural muscles for more effective stabilization.

Anna became a perfect example of my concept of *peeling the onion*. When we started to put things back in place, deeper layers of dysfunction kept coming up to the surface. Her treatment required a long time—more than a year and a half—and included realigning the sacroiliac joint, stretching tight muscles, strengthening weak stabilizers, visceral manipulation, and myofascial techniques, as well as a complete change in her daily yoga practice. Anna then began to heal.

Despite its prevalence as a source of lower back pain, the sacroiliac (SI) is one of the joints most often overlooked by doctors and physical therapists evaluating a person with back pain. In my own experience with yoga practitioners and active young adults, the SI is, more often than not, the cause of chronic and undiagnosed pain and discomfort found in conjunction with lumbar spine dysfunction. Yet because of the complex nature of this joint, it is difficult to identify the type of dysfunction and correct it effectively. In addition, yoga may actually *hurt* more than heal the condition, which is why many yoga practitioners find themselves baffled by pain when they are practicing consistently.

Misalignment of the SI can happen in many directions and can result from trauma or the stress of repetitive movement. Many yoga instructors and practitioners may experience their sacroiliac joints going "out of joint" from asymmetries in their practice as well. Often yoga teachers will demonstrate a pose on the right side and then walk around the room making adjustments on the students, without balancing out their practice on the left side. This, over time, can cause imbalances in the muscles around the hips and pelvis, which can lead to SI joint dysfunction.

In his excellent article "Low back pain's missing link" (2012), John C. Stevenson concludes that:

> up to thirty percent of all low back symptoms are sacroiliac joint in origin, but the diagnosis of a problem with the sacroiliac joint is frequently overlooked because low back pain symptoms have many causes as well as hip joint symptoms. In fact, many patients with disabling low back pain issues go on to receive lumbar spinal treatments and/or hip treatments, although the source of their symptoms may be sacroiliac joint in origin, either in whole or in part, leaving these patients with little or, in some cases, no relief. (p.1)

Understanding sacroiliac joint dysfunction: A joint of stability

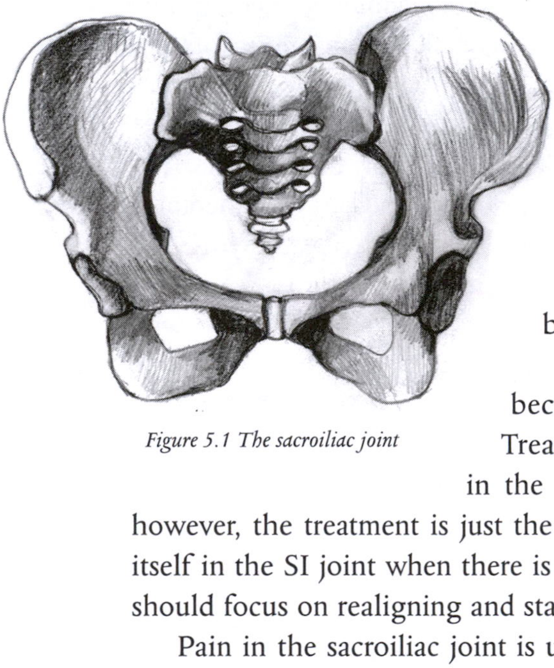

Figure 5.1 The sacroiliac joint

The SI joint is part of the pelvic girdle, and consequently bears the weight of the upper body, translating that weight to the legs via the hip joints. It also is a shock absorber for activities of the lower limbs like running and jumping. Because this area takes the bulk of the weight, it is important that it be strong and stable.

In most other joints, problems emerge because there is not enough mobility. Treatment encourages increasing movement in the joint. When dealing with SI joint pain, however, the treatment is just the opposite. Discomfort will usually present itself in the SI joint when there is *too much* mobility. Treatment in such cases should focus on realigning and stabilizing the joint.

Pain in the sacroiliac joint is usually felt in a localized spot much lower than the lumbar spine—in the area of the dimples of the buttocks. It is usually a sharp pain that worsens with certain movements, either spinal flexion or extension. (In my experience, it is often worse in extension, while flexion relieves the pain. By contrast, disc problems in the lumbar spine feel worse in flexion and better with extension.) Sometimes the pain radiates into the buttocks and can travel to the anterior groin area as well.

In women, the pain can get worse before menstruation as the ligaments that normally hold the SI joint in place may be looser with hormonal fluctuations. Similarly, during pregnancy, women will complain of pain in this area and difficulty walking. This is because hormonal changes have enhanced the mobility of the sacroiliac joint in order to facilitate childbirth.

The sacrum connects to the upper part of both pelvic bones via the SI joints and also to the lumbar spine via the L5–S1 joint (see Figure 5.1). Because of its direct attachment to the lumbar spine, there needs to be some movement in these joints so they can respond directly to movement in the spine. But this flexibility must be balanced by the joint's basic stability.

Normal movements of the sacrum are called *nutation* and *counternutation*. What this means, in simple terms, is that the top of the sacrum moves in the *opposite* direction to the lumbar spine. This is a movement that happens *automatically* in a healthy joint and is beyond our control. Nutation refers to the top of the sacrum tipping forward as a reaction to extension (back bends) in the lumbar spine. Counternutation is when the top of the sacrum tips backward as a reaction to spinal flexion (forward bends) (see Figure 5.2). It is important, as yoga teachers, students, and therapists, to become familiar with these two subtle movements that are present in the sacroiliac joint. Consider the practice tip below for an experiential exercise for you and your clients.

a.
b.

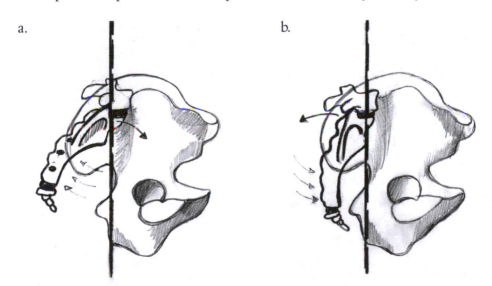

Figure 5.2 Movement in the sacroiliac joint: a. nutation; b. counternutation

PRACTICE TIP 12

Sit on the ground or on a cushion with your legs crossed.

Place your right hand on your sacrum with your fingers pointing down. Slowly arch your back, moving into a slight back bend in the lumbar spine as you shift the weight into the front of your sitting bones. See if you can feel the top of the sacrum move into the body as the lumbar spine moves into extension (see Figure 5.3).

Next, move into a forward bend by shifting the weight back into the sitting bones and rounding the lower back. With the heel of the hand on top of the sacrum, feel the sacral base move backwards, away from the body, in conjunction with lumbar flexion.

Now try to work on a deeper back bend such as Ustrasana/camel pose, as well as a deeper forward bend like Paschimottanasana/seated forward fold, with your hand on the sacrum. See if you can feel the movement of nutation and counternutation in these poses.

a. 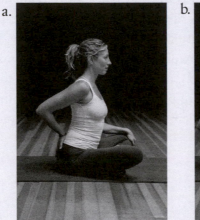 b.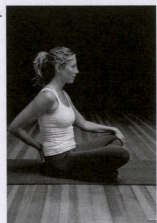

Figure 5.3 Experiential exercise to feel nutation and counternutation of the sacroiliac joint: a. lumbar extension with consequent nutation in SI joint; b. lumbar flexion with counternutation in the SI joint

Because the nature of SI dysfunction can vary from one person to the next, *pushing through SI pain is never recommended.* Your student or client will need to have the sacrum realigned by a professional (physical therapist, osteopath, or chiropractor) so that normal movement can be restored. In addition to having the sacrum realigned, they will need to identify the tight muscles and weak muscles that contribute to this dysfunction so that it does not recur.

Once the SI joint is realigned, the work of their yoga practice will be to stabilize the joint in its proper position. You will want to guide your students to move with control in all postures, focusing on strength rather than flexibility, on *containment and restraint,* rather than opening. This is hard for most yoga practitioners, since the emphasis is often placed on going deeper into poses.

Yoga, and especially therapeutic Purna Yoga in this case, means backing off and creating stability where there was none, a task that is difficult not only for the physical body but also for the ego. Tell your students or clients that if they find themselves bumping up against their will to do more than they should, to go farther than is healthy for them, they are most likely frustrated, but on the right track!

Asanas to help with SI joint pain

Initially, you should recommend postures that relieve tension around the SI joint. You can guide your students or clients through the following postures that tend to create some space and provide relief from inflammation and pain in the initial phases of injury.

1. Purna Yoga Low Back Series

This series from Chapter 3 will help release tension in the spinal muscles, the psoas, and the myofascial complex around the pelvis and sacrum.

2. Half forward bend (Ardha Uttanasana)

Stand facing the wall and place your hands at approximately waist height against the wall. Walk back slowly so that your arms are straight as you press into the wall with your palms. Take your feet wide so that they are in line with the outer edges of your mat, and make sure your feet are directly underneath your hips. Turn the toes in slightly so that your feet are slightly pigeon toed.

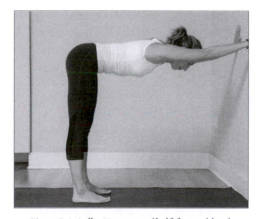

Figure 5.4 Ardha Uttanasana/half forward bend

Contract the quadriceps strongly, lifting the kneecaps up as you press the tops of the thighs back. Take the inner thighs back as you focus on widening the sacroiliac joint. Move the pelvis away from the rib cage as you press into the wall with your hands, creating traction in your lower back. Lift the pit of the abdomen so that you do not collapse into your lower back. Hold for 30 seconds. Repeat two to three times.

3. Cross straps

With wall ropes: Place two straps at waist height, or at the middle rung, in the yoga wall. Cross the straps and step into the loops, one leg at a time, facing away from the yoga wall. Place the straps in the hip creases and lean forward, bringing your hands to the ground. Walk your feet back to the wall and place the heels up the wall. Walk your hands forward so that you are in downward-facing dog position.

a.

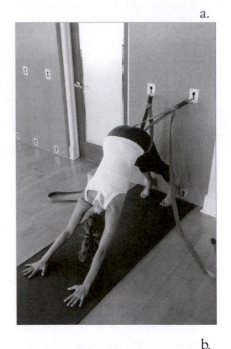

While in the position, focus on the internal rotation of the top of the thighs, as in Exercise 2 above, while spreading the sacroiliac joint open.

With yoga strap on doorknob: If you do not have access to a yoga wall, this is a nice alternative that gives you a similar effect. Secure the yoga strap around your waist, placing the strap at the top of the sacrum. Then take the front of the strap through your legs and loop it over a strong doorknob. Walk forward to create some tension in the strap, and place your hands on the floor. Then walk your feet back so that you are in a supported downward-facing

b.

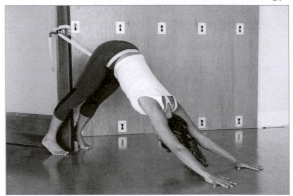

Figure 5.5 a. Cross straps with the yoga wall; b. cross straps without the yoga wall

dog position with support in both your hip creases. While in the position, focus on the internal rotation of the top of the thighs, as in Exercise 2, while spreading the SI joint open. Hold for 30 seconds to one minute. Repeat two to three times. It is all right for the heels to come off the floor in this position, although you want to work towards the heels touching the floor for greater hamstring opening.

The next exercises tend to focus on stabilization of the SI joint complex:

4. SI stabilization with two straps

Place two yoga belts around your hips. Make sure the straps are low, so that they are secured around your pelvis, and are *not* on the waist.

Tighten the straps, with the buckles in the back. Make sure the straps are fastened in opposite directions for maximum stability. You can practice yoga with the straps in this position, or you can wear them throughout the day if you need extra stability. This should feel good on your SI joint and provide immediate relief. If it does not relieve pain or discomfort, do not do the exercise.

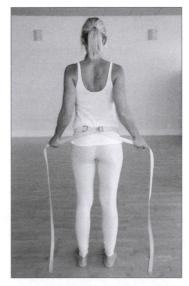

Figure 5.6 Placement of straps around pelvis to increase SI stability

5. Tadasana (mountain pose) with block

Stand in Tadasana (as described in Chapter 3).

- Place a block between your upper thighs and stand with your feet hips' distance apart. This provides a stable base of support in line with the pelvis.

- Press all four corners of your feet into the earth, lifting the arches. This proper contact with the ground energizes the leg muscles and prevents pronation (flat feet) and supination (arched feet) of the feet, so that the hips and knees are in proper alignment. In addition, the more you ground into the earth, the more you will lengthen, so think about *rooting* in order to *lift*.

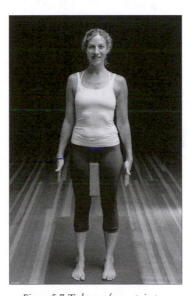

Figure 5.7 Tadasana/mountain pose

- Engage your quadriceps by lifting your kneecaps up into your thighs. It is essential to fire the quadriceps in standing so that the legs hold the weight of the body, not the lower back, which is the more vulnerable part.

- Squeeze the block with your inner thighs and try to push the block out the back. Relax your buttocks. This will create a subtle internal rotation

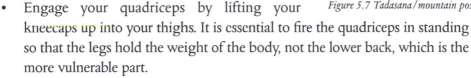

action in the hip joint, which helps to relax the powerful gluteus maximus muscle and opens up the sacroiliac joint and lower back.

- Maintaining the internal rotation, locate your lower belly (the area between the navel and the pubic bone) and lift your lower belly towards your head. This action is very important for maintaining length in the lower back, as well as stabilizing the core. As you lift the pit of the abdomen (POA), you can feel your sacrum descending towards the earth. *Avoid tucking,* as this creates a posterior pelvic tilt—which puts excessive pressure on the discs and vertebrae, since the natural curve of the lower back is lost. In addition, tucking occurs with a strong contraction of the buttocks, which creates more tension in your lower back and sacroiliac joint.

- Move your shoulder blades away from your ears and lift your sternum. When you descend the shoulder blades, it helps to open your chest and relax the upper trapezius (neck) muscle.

- Lengthen through the crown of the head. This creates length through the entire spine from the inside out and prevents a forward head posture. Hold this pose, focusing on all of the above instructions, for one to two minutes. Release and repeat two times every hour.

6. Wall squat with block

- Stand against a wall with the back of your head, upper back, and sacrum touching the wall. Remember it is normal for the lower back to have a natural curve, so it will not touch the wall.

- Slide down the wall into a small squat (never bring the hips below the knees, as it creates tension on the knees).

- Place a block between your thighs and squeeze the block as you hold this position for 30 seconds to one minute. Repeat two to three times.

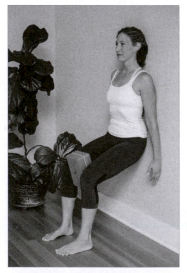

Figure 5.8 Wall squat with a block

7. Bridging with block

Lie on your back and bring your heels close to your buttocks.

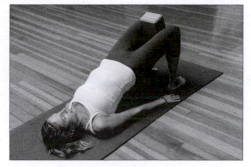

Figure 5.9 Bridging with a block

- Place a block between your thighs so that the thighs are hips' distance apart, and squeeze the block. While squeezing the block, press your feet into the ground and use the leg muscles to lift your hips up.

- Never roll the shoulders away from the ears in this pose. Instead, roll them under the body but do *not* move them away from the ears. Hold a strap or clasp your hands behind your back, pressing your forearms, wrists, and hands into the ground.

- Lift the pit of the abdomen and press the outer shoulders into the ground to open the chest.

- Do not let the block drop, by keeping the inner thighs activated for the duration of the pose.

- Hold for 30 seconds to one minute. Repeat two to three times.

8. Advanced bridging on therapy ball

As you get stronger, you can begin to challenge yourself with a therapy ball.

- *Bridging with both legs on a ball:* Place both calves on the ball as you lie on your back with the arms by your side. Press your hands into the ground and lift your hips up, trying to prevent the ball from moving underneath your legs. Hold here for five seconds and release slowly. Do three sets of ten repetitions.

- *Bridging with one leg on a ball:* Cross your left foot over your right ankle and repeat the exercise above. This will force you to use the right side of your pelvis more, and will increase the work for the stabilizers due to decreased balance. Repeat for right foot over left ankle. Do one to three sets of ten repetitions.

If there is any pain or discomfort, discontinue this exercise. Remember, this is for advanced strengthening once the inflammation has subsided.

a.

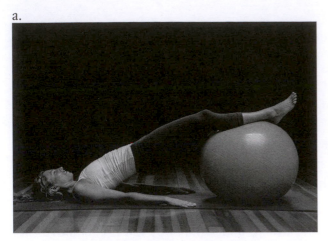

b.

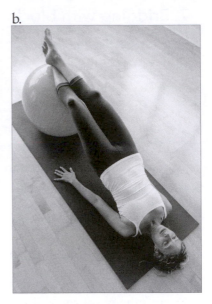

Figure 5.10 a. Bridging on therapy ball;
b. advanced bridging with one leg

9. Supported Halasana (plow pose)

One of my favorite poses that relieves tension in the lower back and SI joint even after the most vigorous practice is Supported Halasana. You will need a bench or a chair with folded blankets to prepare for this posture.

- Place three blankets with the folded edges stacked on top of each other on your mat.

- Rest your shoulders *on* the blankets, while your head rests on the ground (see Figure 5.11 b.). It is important that your lowest cervical vertebra, C7, is resting on the blankets. C7 is one of the first prominent bones that you can feel as you run your fingers down the back of your neck.

- Lift your legs overhead and rest the front top of your thighs on a Halasana bench or chair with blankets, at the level of the hip crease. You should feel that your thighs are being lifted by the bench, and that your pelvis is experiencing traction/lengthening with the support of the bench.

- Take your arms beyond your head and shoulders at 90° and rest them with the elbows bent.

- Hold for five minutes.

- To come out, slowly lower your legs to the ground. Push the bench or chair away from you and slide your shoulders back off the blankets until they reach the floor. Bend your knees and lie here for a few moments, allowing your chest to open as you take a few deep breaths.

- Roll to the side slowly, and press up to a seated position.

a.
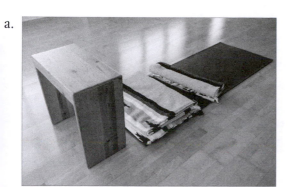

b.
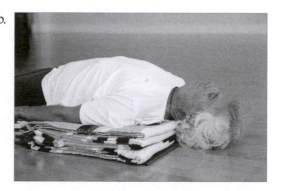

c.
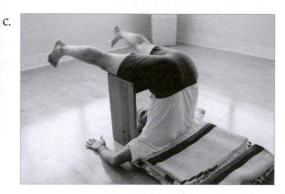

d.
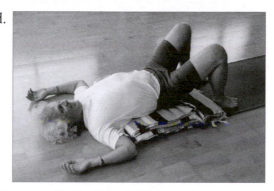

Figure 5.11 a. Halasana set up with props; b. C7 resting on blankets (do not let it slide off when you come into the pose); c. Halasana pose; d. coming out of the pose

10. Legs up the wall with a weight

Lie on your back with your legs up the wall at 90°, keeping your arms at the sides of your body with the palms facing upwards.

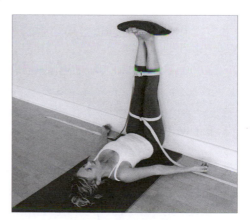

Figure 5.12 Viparita Karani/ legs up the wall with a weight

- Tie a strap around the center of the upper thighs in order to keep the thighs together. (This will help your students relax more fully into the pose, as they do not have to hold their legs up with any effort.)

- You can also tie a second strap around the center of the thighs, fastening it in the opposite direction of the first strap, for added stability.

- Place a ten-pound weight on the soles of the feet for added compression.

- Hold for five minutes.

Healing beyond the postural

As Anna moved from pain and inflammation into stabilization of her SI joints, she began to realize what a highly sensitive person she was. Her nervous system, and therefore her body, was reacting to everything around her. She knew that she had to begin to work on the emotional component of her symptoms, exploring the observation that her pain was relieved when she took a vacation from her husband and her living situation. She admitted to feeling insecure about where she belonged, and longed to live closer to the forest and trees. She did not know where to put her energy and was realizing that she had lost her sense of self and her purpose.

It was clear to me, as well as to others, what a strong, beautiful, and powerful woman she was, but she couldn't see it. She didn't see her power and therefore was unable to stand strong in it.

Anna had to re-evaluate her entire approach to her practice. She learned that she was still looking at yoga in a postural sense, and when she was forced to stop pushing so hard physically, she found herself more open to the introspective parts of yoga. For the first time, she was living her yoga instead of going through the motions.

A few years later, she felt grateful for her injury; it had helped her find her way back to herself. She began to study yoga's sister science of Ayurveda and became a practitioner. Her process of self-exploration allowed her to understand and empathize with others in pain. She made several big decisions. She divorced her husband, and moved to a new city near the trees that she longed for.

She realized that she was hiding behind her physical activities and athleticism, which were simply serving as a distraction from the pain and emptiness she was feeling inside. Instead of being introspective, she would go for a run. She was addicted to endorphins to feel all right in this world, and would move so that she did not have to experience the difficult emotions that would come up when she was not "doing anything."

Anna said, "I used to think that people who don't do things are weak. Now I realize that there's a lot of strength in being able to do nothing."

Anna's healing journey shows how a yoga practice, particularly the intense focus on physical postures alone, can become an escape. It is a healthier addiction than overeating or drugs, but it is an escape nonetheless. Just as I had to change my practice from an aggressive approach to a more thoughtful one, Anna initially moved vigorously in order to quiet her mind, but then had to stop moving so she could start *feeling* in order to heal.

Many clients whom I have seen in my practice with significant SI joint dysfunction present a similar profile to Anna's. They are usually young women who are very fit and active. They may be attractive, carry themselves well, and appear strong and accomplished professionals. On the outside, they have it "all together." In my office, however, once we begin to talk, I can see that their strength and confident exterior is often a response to a very sensitive and fragile interior sense of self that can hinge on the reactions of others around them very easily. Frequently these women admit to having feelings of being "unworthy," of not having been given a strong sense of self by their family of origin, and have difficulty "standing on their own two feet." Consequently, many of these women have also turned towards helping professions to find meaning in their existence. They are teachers, healers, and healthcare workers. Some will describe a feeling that they are not quite fulfilling their purpose (or dharma) in life, but have a hard time taking the leap and believing in their own inner power and resilience.

Your treatment will have to incorporate your client's emotional landscape and belief system in conjunction with their physical (asana) practice and pranayama. You will need to teach them how to focus on stability and rooting in standing poses like Virabhadrasana I and II/warrior I and II, how to trust their inner resilience in Sirsasana/headstand, and how to surrender to their hearts in Sarvangasana/shoulderstand. While working on stability on the physical plane, they will need to explore their ability to "stand on their own two feet" and rest in their inner strength without being swayed by the influence or judgment of others. This is the harder work in the process of yoga therapy, but will lead to a deeper practice and true transformation and healing on all levels.

Getting back to a yoga practice with SI joint instability

Once your student is out of pain, she will need to modify her practice in order to keep the SI joint healthy and to avoid falling back into old patterns of instability. From my experience, a faster-moving vinyasa flow practice tends to aggravate this condition. You will want her to focus on fewer sun salutations and develop a practice that is slower with longer holds. You will also want to make sure her poses are balanced by doing each pose first on the right and then on the left side.

Minimize open pelvis poses like Baddha Konasana/Supta Baddha Konasana (bound angle and reclined bound angle poses) and Virabhadrasana II/warrior II. Instead, work on stability, emphasizing closed pelvis poses like Utkatasana/chair pose, Parsvottanasana/pyramid pose, and Virabhadrasana III/warrior III.

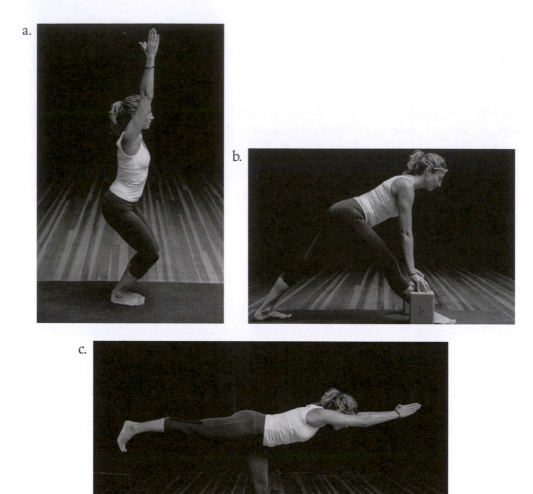

Figure 5.13 a. Utkatasana/chair pose; b. Parsvottanasana/pyramid pose;
c. Virabhadrasana III/warrior III pose

I particularly like two variations of Virabhadrasana III/warrior III that
help to build strength in the stabilizers of the hips and pelvis during this
challenging pose.

1. Warrior III with foot against the wall

- Measure the correct distance from the wall so that your leg can be straight, with the entire sole of the foot pressing firmly into the wall.

- Place a block on the floor in front of you and place your hands on the block as you hinge from the hips to bend forward with a straight spine.

- Draw the shoulder blades away from the ears and take the sternum forward to open the chest.

- *Slowly* lift your right leg off the ground, keeping the toes and knee pointing down towards the ground.

- Rotate the right thigh internally by bringing the inner thigh up towards the sky.

- Lift your leg so it is parallel with your buttocks and place the sole of the foot against the wall.

- Press the foot firmly into the wall and tighten the quadriceps, keeping your back leg perfectly straight.

- Lift the quadriceps in the left leg as well, and lengthen the spine.

- Hold for 30 seconds and repeat on the other side. Repeat two to three times on each side, alternating sides.

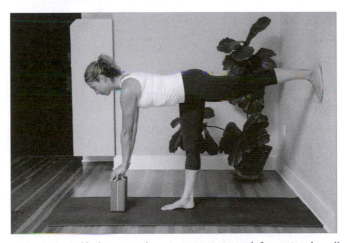

Figure 5.14 Virabhadrasana III/warrior III variation with foot against the wall

2. Half downward-facing dog with hands on the wall

- Come into half downward-facing dog pose, with your arms straight against the wall at about waist level, and feet directly underneath the hips.

- Focus on maintaining internal rotation in your right leg as you *siowly* lift the leg up so it is parallel with the buttocks and spine.

- Drop the right outer hip as you lift the left outer hip, to keep the pelvis level for the duration of the pose.

- Hold for 30 seconds. Repeat two to three times, alternating right and left.

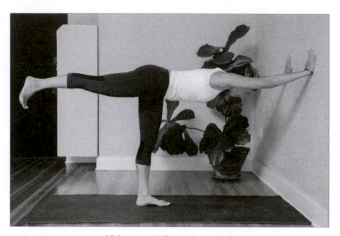

Figure 5.15 Half downward-facing dog with hands on the wall

To summarize, *emphasize strength in your students' postures instead of increasing their flexibility.* Have them back off a little before hitting their edge, and work on hugging the thighs inward towards one another as if they are squeezing a block between their legs in all poses.

You can also have your students practice with two straps, as previously mentioned (see Figure 5.6), which will help maintain stability and decrease pain during any bouts of recurring SI joint pain.

CASE STUDY: MARK

Treatment Session 3

Mark does not have SI joint instability. Instead, like many men, he has *decreased* pelvic mobility and therefore needs to open his SI joint. Sometimes a lack of mobility in the SI joint can create lower back pain, since all the movement in the pelvis is translated to the lumbar spine instead of being distributed evenly among the SI joints and vertebrae. If the movements of *nutation* and *counternutation* are absent in the SI joint, then the whole pelvis is essentially moving as one solid block. For those who move this way, please teach them how to move their pelvis relative to their spine and encourage the natural mobility of the sacroiliac joints.

For Mark's treatment session we focused on:

- cat/cow (Marjarasana) variations on all fours and in sitting, with education about anterior and posterior pelvic tilt

- downward-facing dog on the yoga wall with cross straps to increase space in the SI joint. Mark was encouraged to turn his toes in slightly to help facilitate internal rotation of the thighs. He was then instructed to direct his breath into the SI joint, visualizing the space opening up and expanding with each inhalation, and releasing any tension on the exhalation

- bridging with a block between the legs—to increase strength in the inner thighs and decrease tightness in the outer thighs, to prevent turning out of the legs and create more internal support.

As we move forward with Mark's treatment, we will continue to reinforce increased pelvic mobility throughout each posture.

CHAPTER 6

Creating Space
Traction

Imagine your bones and breath as traincars: no space between them and you are headed for a wreck.

Matthew J. Taylor

People often ask me whether they can ever heal and be pain-free once they have been diagnosed with a spinal condition. They may experience degenerative disc disease, a herniated disc, scoliosis, or stenosis, yet they express the same concerns. They ask, "Won't I always have pain, since there are visible changes on my MRI?" Or, "Aren't those changes irreversible?"

While it is true that changes detected by an MRI may not be reversible and that arthritis does not get better with age, that does not mean their pain cannot be relieved. In fact, many people do return to the activities they enjoyed prior to the onset of their symptoms. How is this possible?

In his *Healing Back Pain* (1991), orthopedic physician John Sarno cites two research studies that explored the relationship between spinal abnormalities and back pain:

> Between 1976 and 1980, two Israeli physicians, Dr. A. Magora and Dr. A. Schwartz, published four medical articles in the *Scandinavian Journal of Rehabilitation* in which they reported the results of studies they had done to determine whether certain spinal abnormalities caused back pain. Their method was to compare the X-rays of people with or without a history of back pain. If people with back pain had these abnormalities more commonly, one could presume that the abnormalities might be the cause of the pain.
>
> They found no statistical difference in the incidence of degenerative osteoarthritis, transitional vertebra, spina bifida occulta, and spondylosis between the two groups. There was a

small statistical significance for spondylolisthesis. In other words, one could not attribute back pain to these disorders, with the possible exception of spondylolisthesis.

A similar study was conducted by American radiologist Dr. C. A. Splithoff and published in the *Journal of the American Medical Association* in 1953. He compared the incidence of nine different abnormalities of the end of the spine in people with and without back pain. Again he found no statistical significance. (Sarno 1991, pp.131–132)

In addition to these studies, Sarno points out that individuals who have back pain are predominantly between the ages of 30 and 60 years old; 77 percent of the incidence is in this age range (pp.5, 6). This is a strange phenomenon, since older individuals, those more than 70 or 80 years of age, often have more degenerative changes than people in the younger age group. From this we can conclude that the severity of degenerative changes in the spine does not necessarily correlate with pain, since the younger group suffers more from back pain than the older group. Because this is the case, we must ask what the real cause of pain is in individuals between the ages of 30 and 60.

Sarno notes that stress and anxiety are highest during the years when we are moving up in our careers, starting and raising families, and experiencing greater financial responsibility. Stress affects the tissues and creates more muscular tension, which, in turn, causes the muscles to clamp down around the vertebrae. When the muscles are tight, there is less space between each vertebra, both in the joint and in the space from which nerves exit from the spinal cord to the limbs. It is, in fact, this compression, this narrowing of the joint space, which creates pain and discomfort.

Even when arthritis and degeneration occur in the spine, as long as the joint surfaces do not touch one another or pinch a nerve, there will not be any pain. Pain is caused by *compression* from either tight muscles or bony changes. When we know that this is the cause, we also know that there is a simple solution to most cases of lower back pain—*traction*.

In the medical field, traction is translated as "a deliberate, sustained pull applied mechanically, especially to the arm, leg, or neck, so as to correct fractured or dislocated bones, overcome muscle spasms, or relieve pressure." In our case, traction refers to creating space between the vertebrae so that joint surfaces do not rub against one another, and there is no compression of surrounding structures. *In most cases, traction is the key to maintaining a Happy Back.*

Often in physical therapy and yoga therapy, traction involves the careful, deliberate, and prolonged lengthening of a muscle or joint, usually by submitting it to the natural force of gravity. The goal of spinal traction is to lengthen the spine and surrounding muscles, thus creating space and decompressing the vertebrae. This, too, is what we ultimately strive for in our yoga practice. If done properly, yoga postures (asana) should decrease weight and compression on the lower back. However, when we practice aggressively or do not learn how to activate the appropriate muscles, the same postures can have the opposite effect. We can actually create more compression in the spine and more tightness in our muscles.

To sum up, the goal of spinal traction is actually twofold: First, we want to release tight muscles around the spine so that the joint space can be increased. Second, we want to relieve compression of—that is, decompress—any structures, especially the nerves, between the vertebrae.

When to avoid traction

Traction is recommended for most back pain except in the acute phase of an injury. When any area of the spine is inflamed, initially it is important to *avoid bilateral traction*. This refers to the movement of both sides of the pelvis away from the lumbar spine at the same time. The reason for this is that, during the initial phases of injury, the spinal muscles naturally contract in order to protect the spine from further movement and, therefore, further injury. If traction is applied during this acute phase of muscle spasm, the affected area may feel good while in traction, because the compression is relieved. But as soon as the traction is released, the muscles will tighten, this time with a vengeance, creating more pain than previously. We must always respect the body's wisdom, but especially during this acute phase of the injury. Therefore the only kind of traction appropriate at this stage is unilateral traction in a neutral position. This safe technique is described below.

Traction techniques

1. Unilateral traction: Safe traction for the acute phase

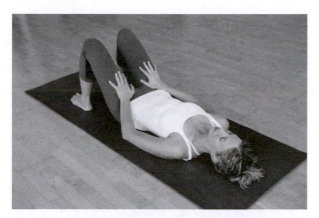

Figure 6.1 Unilateral traction of the lower back

- Lie on your back with your knees bent.

- Place the base of the palms of your hands in your hip creases.

- Take a deep inhalation.

- On the exhalation, press the right palm into the right hip crease, moving the femur bone away from your head. At the same time, lift the pit of the abdomen (POA) towards your head. If you have difficulty lifting the POA, refer back to Chapter 3.

- Relax on the inhalation. On the exhalation, press the palm into the left thigh as you lift the POA.

- Keep alternating legs, pushing the thighs away on each exhalation.

- Repeat 18 times, alternating legs.

When using this preliminary technique, note how the breath must be coordinated with the movement in order for the exercise to have its maximum impact. The student is at rest during the inhalation, and on the exhalation is encouraged to push the thighbone away from her head and lift the pit of the abdomen towards the head. Activation of the abdominal muscles is encouraged by exhalation. This coordination, with the breath leading the movement, must continue as you ease into other forms of traction once the acute pain has subsided.

2. Reclined hand to big toe pose (Supta Padangusthasana) with two straps

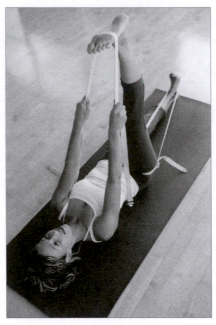

Figure 6.2 Supta Padangusthasana with two straps

- Lie on your back with your left leg extended and your right knee bent.

- Place a yoga strap in the right hip crease, with the buckle facing *away* from your hip and the other end of the strap just above the left heel. Make sure the strap is tight when you lift your right leg up.

- To tighten the strap: bend the left knee, pull the buckle away from the right hip, and then straighten the left leg.

- Keep both thigh muscles contracted and shoulders pressing into the floor.

- Move the right thighbone away from your head, emphasizing creating space in the right hip crease.

- Keep pressing your left heel into the strap, while pressing the left thighbone down into the ground. Hold for one minute.

After you release, you will need to reposition the strap in the left hip crease and on the right heel, and repeat on the left side.

3. Supine traction—with two belts and a block, lying down

This technique is best done with a certified Purna Yoga teacher.

- Place one loop around your waist and fasten over the frontal hipbones (also known as the ASIS—anterior superior iliac spine), with the second strap hanging in the center of your back like a tail (Figure 6.3).

Note: It is important that you place the strap over the pelvic bones (ASIS) at the beginning of the exercise, and not on the waist. By the time the legs are straight, the strap should have slid over the ASIS into the abdomen.

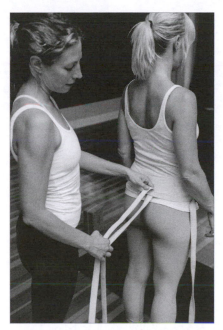

Figure 6.3 Placement of straps on pelvis in standing position

- Lie on your mat, with the strap between your legs in the center.

- Place a block in the loop and place both feet on the block, with your knees bent.

- Straighten your legs by pressing your feet into the block. If it is easy to straighten the legs, tighten the strap one inch and straighten the legs again.

- Continue tightening one inch at a time, until it is so tight that you can just barely straighten your legs and the entire pelvis tips over backwards.

- Once you are in the final position, bend your knees on the inhalation and straighten your legs on the exhalation. Repeat that final pump nine times.

Note: The strap must be just the right length, so that it is difficult to straighten the legs with the knees fully extended. This will provide resistance and the force necessary to create traction in your lower back.

• When you have completed the repetitions, roll over to the side and stay there for a few breaths before pushing up to a seated position.

a.
b.
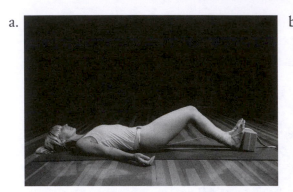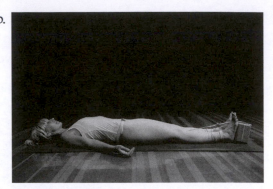

Figure 6.4 a. Supine position with feet on block; b. final pose with legs pressing into block

• Next, stand up *with the straps on your pelvis*, and begin to walk around the room. This will teach your body how to maintain a state of traction afterwards, and will prevent muscle spasm. Walk with the straps on for one minute.

• Gently remove the straps and begin to walk around the room again, allowing your body to feel the effects of the pose. Continue walking around for three to five minutes.

4. Downward-facing dog/Adho Mukha Svanasana on the door with cross stretch, twist, and assisted

This posture is one of the best ways to create traction in the lower back. Gravity assists the lengthening, while breath and awareness facilitate it. It is also fun! The posture can be done on a door hinge or, preferably, with two yoga straps and a block.

Set-up 1

• Loop two straps together making one longer strap.

• Place the end of the strap over a strong door hinge—in the opposite direction as the door would open—and feed the strap through, fastening it into a large circle.

• Adjust the strap so that it is roughly at the level of the hip creases.

- You will need to readjust as necessary so that the heels can touch the door, while the arms are outstretched on the ground, with the head 3–6 inches off the floor.

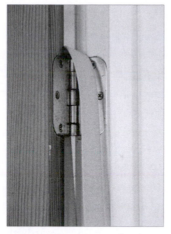

Figure 6.5 Set-up 1 on a door hinge

Set-up 2

- Loop two straps together to make one big circle.

- Place a block in the circle and feed the block over the door, in the center, in the opposite direction of opening.

- Then close the door, testing the block to make sure that it is stable and can hold your weight on the strap.

- Adjust the strap so that it is roughly at the level of the hip creases.

- As above, you will need to readjust as necessary so that your heels can touch the door, while your arms are outstretched on the ground, with your head 3–6 inches off the floor.

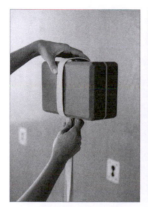
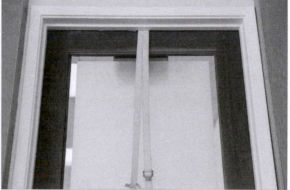

Figure 6.6 Set-up 2 with a block in the center of the door (preferred)

Now you should be set up in a supported downward-facing dog/Adho Mukha Svanasana position, with your heels up the door and toes away from the door. Once in the pose you can practice three different variations of traction, listed below.

a. Hanging dog

- Place your feet hips' distance apart and make sure that your feet are pointing straight ahead. Align the outer edges of the feet with the edges of your mat.

- Engage your thigh muscles as you extend your knees, feeling as if you are drawing the kneecaps up into the thighbones. Avoid "locking the knees" by pushing the knees back, and rather focus on the lift in the frontal thighs towards the hip crease or groin area.

- Take the skin of the inner thighs back towards the door in order to create a sense of spreading in the lower back and sacroiliac joint. This action can also be described as slight internal rotation of the thighs.

- Walk your hands out in front of you and make sure the hands are both level. (This is especially helpful for individuals with scoliosis, as one side of their spine will be shorter than the other. In this case, we will work on lengthening the shorter side by walking the hand forward to meet the opposite side. This will start to create length and balance to the spinal curves.)

- Take a deep inhalation.

- As you exhale, stretch out through the fingertips and lengthen the whole spine forward, beginning from the lower back/lumbar spine.

- Keep the lower belly slightly engaged to protect the lower back.

- Relax the head and neck.

- Hold here for one to two minutes.

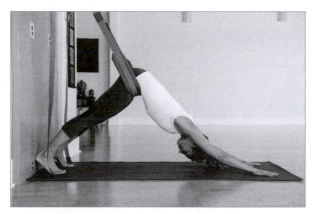

Figure 6.7 Downward-facing dog / Adho Mukha Svanasana with traction

b. Cross stretch

- Starting in hanging dog, bend the right knee and stretch out through the right fingertips on the exhalation.

- Inhaling, straighten the right leg.

- On the next exhalation, bend the left knee and stretch out through the left fingertips.

- Continue this pattern, alternating lengthening each side, three to five times.

- This variation will encourage more lengthening on one side. *If your student has one side that is tighter than the other, you can instruct her to do twice as many repetitions on the limited side.*

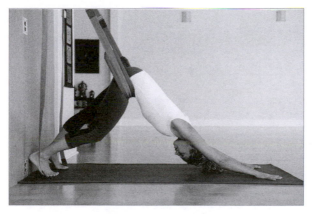

Figure 6.8 Cross stretch

c. Downward-facing dog with a twist

- Take hold of the outside of your left thigh, shinbone, or ankle (for those who are more flexible) with your right hand, placing the left hand on the floor to the side, with the elbow bent.

- Keep your lower belly engaged to protect the lower back, and relax your head and neck.

- Take a deep breath in, and on the exhalation pull the outer ankle (thigh or shinbone) with your right hand, and twist throughout the whole spine.

- Release on the inhalation.

- Take your left hand to the right outer thigh, shinbone, or ankle (keep it the same as the right side for balance) and place your right hand on the ground with the elbow bent.

- On the exhalation, pull your outer right leg with your left hand as you twist throughout the spine.

Note: Most of the rotation should come from your thoracic spine, not the lumbar area. Encourage your students to move from the area in between the shoulder blades with verbal or manual cues. This pose is also a fantastic chest opener and stretches out the pectoral muscles in the anterior chest.

This is a wonderful way to incorporate twisting into your program. This particular version of the pose "lengthens the spine" as you twist, an action impossible to do when done right side up. The spine naturally shortens during all twists. Doing twists with the help of gravity and traction enables your students to receive the benefits of twisting without the risk of compression.

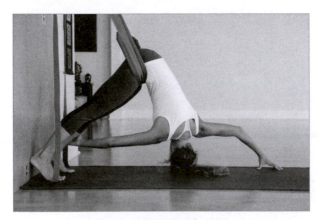

Figure 6.9 Traction with a twist

As you can see, there are many variations to accomplishing traction in your lower back. With each technique it is important to visualize the area of tightness, move breath into that area, and then exhale as you release tension.

In addition, there are many more possibilities for achieving the benefits of traction if you work with the yoga wall, and I highly encourage therapists and teachers who work with spinal conditions to purchase a wall for classes and private sessions. The next section will focus on postures that can be done using The Great Yoga Wall™ or any similar tractioning device.

For teachers with a yoga wall
Pelvic swing with breath and awareness

This technique is one of the best ways to invite students to start to release tension in their spinal muscles in order to facilitate traction of the lumbar spine. It also provides them with immediate feedback on the quality of lengthening they can experience. This pose is best practiced on a yoga wall for safety.

- Be certain that the pelvic swing is at the level of the hip creases and not on the top of the thighs when coming into this position. If there is any pain in the thigh muscles, have the student come down and reposition the swing so it rests higher up in the hips.

- Next, the student should lean forward, place the hands on the floor, and walk the feet up the wall so that the feet are slightly below hip level. Make sure the feet are roughly hips' distance apart and the toes are pointing down towards the floor.

- The head should be off the ground (at least six inches).

- The backs of the hands should rest on the floor with the palms facing upward so that the upper back can remain relaxed.

Note: It is very helpful to measure the distance from the crown of the head to the floor for reference. It is a nice tool to have in order to show your client how much length they have gained by hanging with the help of gravity and the breath.

- Take a deep inhalation, feeling the breath move into the lower back area.

- Ask the student to exhale and visualize the lumbar vertebrae moving away from the sacrum: imagine the muscles between the vertebrae lengthening, increasing the intervertebral space.

- Then invite the student to slowly release, vertebra by vertebra, with awareness, starting from the lower lumbar spine and moving up to the base of the neck.

- The instructor should place the fingertips of the first three fingers on the spine; this gives the student manual feedback at each level while he or she focuses on exhaling and releasing the tension in the spinal muscles. Encourage the student to breathe into your fingers, and on the exhalation, release tension from this area.

- Hold for 10 to 20 breaths.

- When the release is complete, measure the distance from the crown of the head to the floor and notice if your spine gained some length!

a.
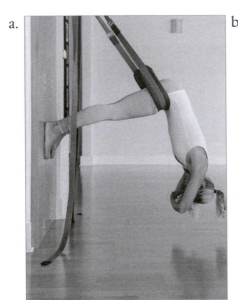
b.
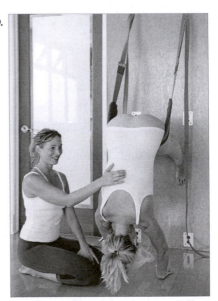

Figure 6.10 a. Full traction on pelvic swing; b. with assistance

Purna Yoga Reversing the Aging of the Spine Series

This sequence was designed by my teacher, Aadil Palkhivala, and incorporates traction with all of the available ranges of motion in the spine—namely, flexion, extension, lateral flexion, and rotation. Instead of asking a student or client to simply hang with gravity to create space, this sequence increases mobility in the spine, while maintaining space between the joints.

Please note: This sequence is for overall spinal health and is especially useful to prevent and help with degenerative disc disease and arthritis. The sequence may have to be modified for those with spinal injuries. Such individuals should practice this sequence with a certified Purna Yoga instructor, and with the approval of their physician.

Contraindications: High blood pressure, stroke, glaucoma, recent eye surgery, and menstruation, due to inversions being practiced.

1. Hanging traction

Begin the sequence with this posture, as described above in pelvic swing (see Figure 6.10 a.).

2. Traction with a twist

In order to teach this variation you will need two straps on the lower rung in addition to the pelvic swing.

- Have the student hang in spinal traction first, then reach with the right hand for the left strap, and place the left hand on the floor with the elbow bent upwards towards the ceiling and fingertips on the floor, facilitating a twist to the left.

- Instruct the student to take a deep breath in, and on the exhalation draw the belly button in towards the spine, pull with both hands, and twist to the left.

- Release gently on the inhalation and pull and twist on the exhalation. Repeat one more time for a total of three rotations to the left. Then release completely.

- Guide the student to use the left arm and take hold of the lower strap on the right, and place the right arm out in front, resting the weight on the fingertips. Have the student inhale and pull while twisting to the right, drawing the navel towards the spine during the twist (this helps protect the lower back while twisting).

- Repeat three times, increasing the rotation in the spine each time as tolerated.

Note: Most of the twisting should be in the upper back. There is a small amount of rotation available in the lower back as well, but the primary focus should be on opening up the chest and thoracic spine.

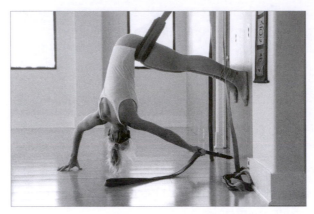

Figure 6.11 Twist on yoga wall with traction

Teacher adjustment: To facilitate more rotation, you can stand at a 45° angle to the student and place your foot out in front of you in the same direction as the twist. The student can then hold onto your ankle as you take them deeper into a twist. The student does most of the work; you simply help take them a little further, being mindful of opening the chest according to the student's limitations. You can run your hands down the length of the spine as the student pulls and twists, emphasizing maintaining length in the spine during the twist.

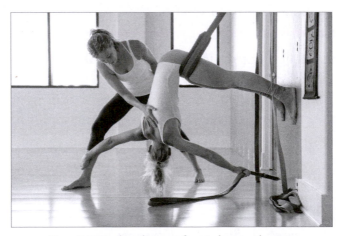

Figure 6.12 Teacher adjustment for spinal twist with traction

3. Lateral flexion with traction

- Again, begin this sequence with the student in hanging traction.

- Invite the student to walk both hands over to the right side, and place the right hand on top of the left one so that the left side of the body is lengthened in the shape of a half moon.

- Ask the student to inhale into the left side of the body, and as the student exhales, instruct her to shift the weight of the hips to the left, increasing the stretch on the left side of the body.

- Repeat three times, increasing the stretch on each exhalation. Release, and repeat on the opposite side by walking the hands out to the left side and placing the left hand over the right. Hold for three breaths.

- Practice three repetitions on each side for three breaths, alternating sides.

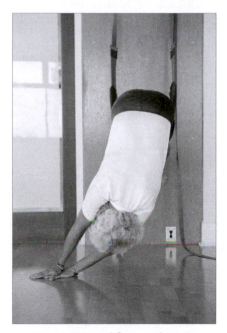

Figure 6.13 Lateral flexion with traction

Teacher adjustment: Stand at a 90° angle to the student, with your right leg in front of you. Have the student take hold of your right ankle with their left hand, and place their right hand just above your knee on your anterior thigh. Stabilize the student's pelvis by placing your right hand on the outer pelvis. Walk backwards, increasing the stretch on the left side of the body as tolerated by your student. Instruct the student to take a deep breath in, and as they exhale have them pull your ankle with their left hand as they push into your knee with their right hand. Repeat three times, with the effort on the exhalation. After three breaths, have the student release, and move to the other side.

Ask the student to hold your left ankle with their right hand and place their left hand above your knee. Walk backwards until the student feels a stretch on the right side of the torso. Then have them pull with the bottom hand and push with the top hand on the exhalations for three breaths. Again, practice three repetitions on each side for three breaths, alternating sides.

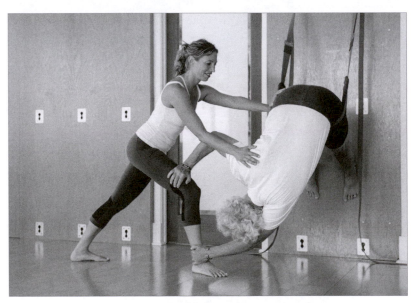

Figure 6.14 Lateral flexion with traction, assisted

4. Spinal extension with traction—with help of a teacher only

Place a "Keeper" (Figure 6.15) around the straps of the pelvic swing to keep the swing together. *Spinal extension should be omitted for anyone with spinal stenosis/spondylolisthesis and if it creates **any** pain in the lumbar spine.*

- Have the student stand in the pelvic swing, facing the wall. Place the pelvic swing *below the lower back, on the sacrum and pelvic bones.* (If the swing slides up too high it can create too much extension in the lumbar spine. The aim is for the pelvic swing to pull the pelvis away from the head, decompressing the spine and aiding traction during spinal extension.)

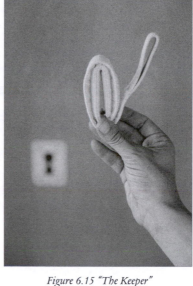

Figure 6.15 "The Keeper"

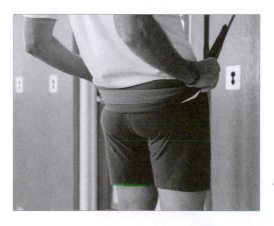

Figure 6.16 Positioning of pelvic swing during spinal extension

- Ask the student to walk their feet up the wall, keeping the feet below the level of the sacrum. Readjust the strap as needed, so that it is over the sacrum and pelvis and not in the arch of the lumbar spine.

- Guide the student to lower down slowly backwards and reach overhead for your waist with both arms. (More flexible students can walk their hands down the teacher's back and reach for the back of the teacher's thighs.)

- Have the student draw the navel strongly towards the spine *on the exhalation* in order to protect the lower back. Remind the student to focus on lengthening the spine at each level as she moves into a gravity-assisted back bend.

- Encourage the student to hold for ten breaths and, with your help around their neck and head, come up slowly.

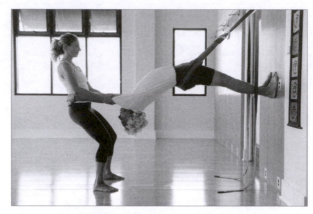

Figure 6.17 Assisted spinal extension with the pelvic swing

Teacher adjustment: Begin by having the student hold onto your waist. Place your hands close to their shoulder joints and assist the student by rolling the upper arm bones outward (into external rotation). As you facilitate chest opening, lean backwards, creating traction in the spine for a more expansive back bend.

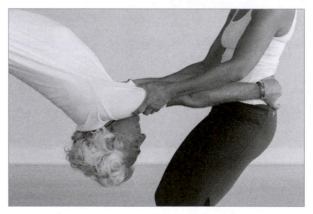

Figure 6.18 Adjustment of upper arms during spinal extension

5. Spinal flexion with traction

This exercise requires the assistance of an instructor in order to support the head. *Omit for disc herniation or bulge and osteoporosis.*

This variation requires two straps in the middle rung of the wall.

- Help the student into a hanging traction position and ask them to reach for the two straps with both hands.

- On the exhalation, the student should pull into a forward bend with the arms, bending the elbows outward as the head moves towards the shinbones.

Teacher adjustment: At this point, you will lie underneath the student on your back and place your hands under the back of their skull in order to support the weight of the head. *Do not press the student's head forward!* Simply support the weight of the head at the point where the student reaches on her own. Instruct the student to rest the weight of their head into your hands so there is no tension in the neck muscles. Then ask the student to relax the upper back and round the area between the shoulder blades towards the floor.

The intention of this technique is to release tension in the upper back area (thoracic spine) and create a natural curve (kyphosis) in this area. This is especially helpful for individuals with a flattened or decreased thoracic curve.

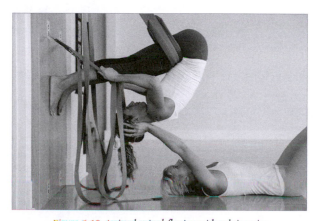

Figure 6.19 Assisted spinal flexion with pelvic swing

Upright traction

For those who may not be able to practice such inversions, you may help them experience traction while upright. This can be done at a yoga wall with the two straps at the highest level. You can also hang from a trapeze-like bar. I often instruct people to find monkey bars in a park to simulate this on their own.

The Purna Yoga Standing Traction Series is outlined below.

Purna Yoga Standing Traction Series

1. Straight traction

- Have the student hold onto the straps (with straps around the wrists) or bar, with the palms facing forward.

- Guide the student to sit down, keeping their back against the wall for support.

- Ensure that the shoulders are kept in joint, and that the focus is on lengthening between the armpits and the hips.

- Suggest that the pelvis feels very heavy as the weight of the lower body releases towards the ground on every exhalation.

- Hold for ten deep breaths.

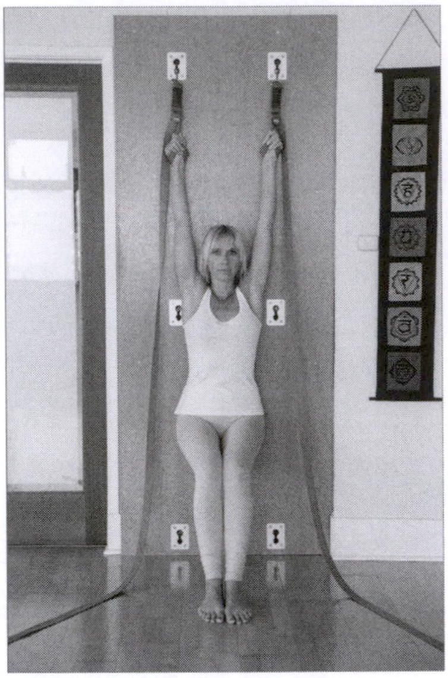

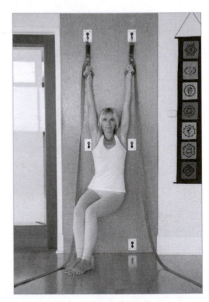

Figure 6.20 Upright traction on yoga wall

2. Pelvic rotation

- Repeat as in straight traction, this time having the student walk the feet towards the right, keeping the knees together for stability.

- On the exhalation, ask your student to focus on dropping the left side of the pelvis down towards the ground to facilitate traction with a twist. Suggest imagining the pelvis moving further away from the rib cage with each breath.

- After a few deep breaths, guide the student to walk the feet to the left and drop the right pelvis down.

- The hold should be five to ten breaths on each side, with a release as needed.

Figure 6.21 Upright traction with a twist

3. Lateral flexion

This posture is excellent for scoliosis, especially on the shortened side (concave side) of the curve, and should be practiced twice as much on the restricted side for individuals with an imbalance.

- Begin as in straight traction and have the student walk both feet out to the side and stack one foot directly on top of the other foot, creating a half-moon shape with the side of the body. Rest the spine against the wall for support.

- Ask the student to move with total awareness, and sink the pelvis down towards the earth, keeping the shoulders in joint and lengthening the side of the waist and armpit area.

- Have the student hold here for ten breaths as tolerated.

- If the student complains of too much pressure on the hands and wrists, suggest that they cross the top leg over the bottom one and rest the foot on the floor (as in Figure 6.22 b.) for added support.

a. b.

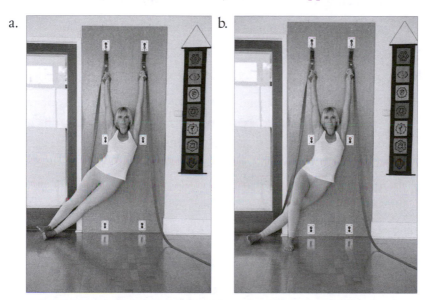

Figure 6.22 a. Upright traction with lateral flexion; b. with leg crossed over for extra support

Other poses that create traction

1. Half forward fold (Ardha Uttanasana) with rope wall and manual traction

This can be done with two assistants or with a yoga wall and one assistant.

- Place the yoga strap in the middle rung and take it over the student's body so that the strap is directly in the hip creases.

- Instruct the student to walk forward until the strap is taut. Make sure that the feet are hips' distance apart and facing forward.

- Have the student reach for the assistant's wrists with the hands, while coming down into a tabletop position with the spine parallel to the floor.

- Ask the student to engage the thighs and lift the kneecaps by contracting the quadriceps muscles. There should be a slight internal rotation of the inner thighs as well.

- Ensure that the student's shoulders remain in joint as the assistant walks backwards, creating traction in the student's spine.

- Encourage focus on lengthening from the armpit towards the top of the pelvis.

- Hold for 30 seconds to a minute and release slowly.

This same effect can be accomplished with two assistants in a class or private setting. One assistant can act as the yoga wall, and places the strap in the hip crease. With the elbows bent and placed alongside the waist, the assistant should lean back, pulling the student's pelvis away from the rib cage. The second assistant should hold onto the student's forearms as in the previous example, and pull the rib cage away from the pelvis (see Figure 6.23 b.).

a. 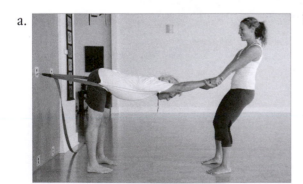   b.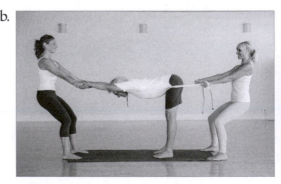

Figure 6.23 a. Half forward fold / Ardha Uttanasana with traction on yoga wall; b. with two assistants

2. Half-pyramid pose (Ardha Parsvottanasana) with rope wall and manual traction

- Set the student up as in the previous pose, but with the right leg forward a few feet.

- Step the left leg back and turn the left foot out at a 45° angle.

- Ask the student to keep both legs perfectly straight and to make the pelvis level. In order to do this, the right outer hip should move away from the strap, and the left outer hip should drop down towards the floor.

- The right big toe mound presses firmly into the earth as the student draws the right outer hip back. This should intensify the stretch behind the right thigh and knee (hamstrings).

- The student can do this on their own, with hands on blocks (as in Figure 6.24), or for more traction they can hold onto the assistant's wrists and keep the shoulders in joint as the assistant pulls back gently. This is important, so as not to strain the shoulders and to feel the traction in the desired area, the spine. As in the previous example, this pose can also be done with two assistants instead of the yoga wall.

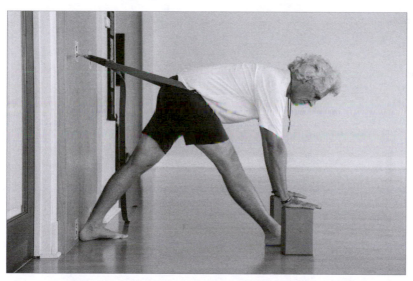

Figure 6.24 Half-pyramid/Ardha Parsvottanasana with traction on yoga wall

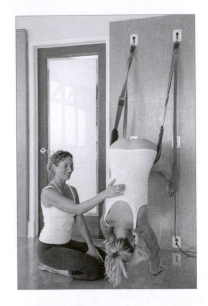

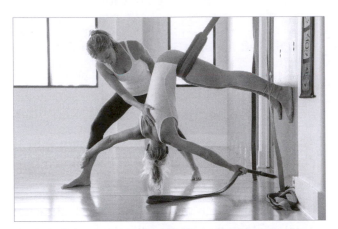

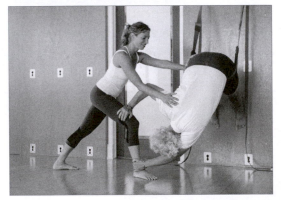

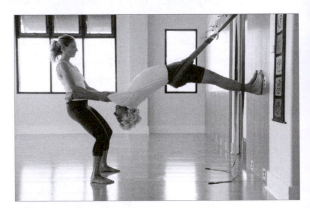

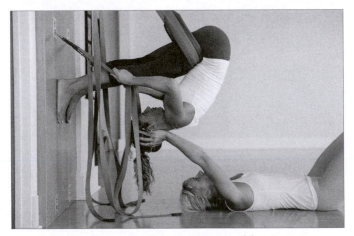

Figure 6.25 Purna Yoga Reversing the Aging of the Spine Series

CASE STUDY: MARK

Treatment Session 4

In the last few sessions with Mark, we have focused on teaching him foundational postural alignment, opening up his hips and increasing pelvic mobility. Now we are ready to introduce traction so that we can help loosen up his back muscles and decompress his spine.

Because his hips are now more open, he is able to go into a supported downward-facing dog position on the door, but he will bend his knees slightly so that his lower back can maintain its natural curve (see Figure 6.26).

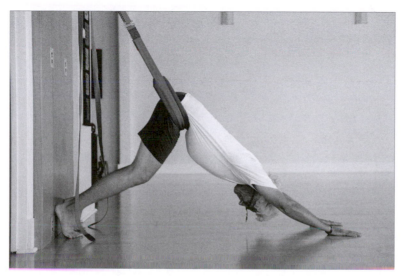

Figure 6.26 Supported downward-facing dog with bend in the knees
(in order to maintain the natural curve of the lower back)

The poses we will work on in this session are:
- hamstring stretch (Supta Padangusthasana) with two belts
- downward-facing dog (Adho Mukha Svanasana) on the yoga wall
- cross stretch
- hanging traction with manual feedback.

In all of these postures we encourage Mark to learn how to introduce the breath into his lower back so that he can release tension on each exhalation. He is accustomed to holding his breath, as well as holding tension in his back and neck, so this is the most challenging part for him. He feels as if he must always be in control, both at work and at home. He feels he never really has the chance to let go. He admits that it is very hard for him to relax and that an element of fear comes up at the thought of being vulnerable.

We talk about this and I assure him that he is safe when he lets go of some of the control during our session. We start with learning how to use breath and body awareness to release tension, for at this point it is safer and more comfortable for Mark to relate to his physical body first.

We will explore his emotional landscape and introduce more tools to address this important element as we move ahead in our treatments together, and as I gain his trust and confidence.

CHAPTER 7

What is the Core Exactly?

Abdominal Strengthening and Back Pain

**Yoga is not about the shape of your body,
but the shape of your life.**

Aadil Palkhivala

As a yoga teacher, therapist, or practitioner, you must have heard the term "core strengthening." In fact, core strength is now a household word and everyone seems to be searching for new ways to obtain a stronger core, which usually equates in their minds with more chiseled abs. This "core" of the body remains mysterious, as there is no clarity about which muscles should be considered a part of this area. And even more mysterious is the certainty with which nearly everyone feels that abdominal strengthening is of paramount importance for individuals with back pain when, in truth, as Lederman has argued in "The myth of core stability" (2007), there is little evidence to support this claim.

Many back pain sufferers are instructed by their healthcare providers as well as their friends to "strengthen the core." Beyond those words, however, there are few guidelines given to these same patients about how to actually accomplish this. Consequently, many individuals begin practicing sit-ups or an array of abdominal exercises they learned at the gym without adequate awareness. Often they harm their spine more than helping it.

If we go back to the five stages of healing presented in Chapter 1, we can see that strength and stabilization is the *fourth* step on the list. There is a good reason for this. We often jump towards strengthening before actually realigning the body. It does not help us to be strong if we continue to experience compression in the spine. Ask your students or clients: would they fortify and paint the walls of a house whose foundation is falling apart?

If the foundation is crooked, all the "external" work will go to waste, as the structure will eventually collapse from within. We can always build a new house, but when it comes to our bodies, we each have one that must last a lifetime. As therapists and teachers, we must persuade our clients and students that it is worth the investment it takes to align the internal structure, their foundation, namely the pelvis and spine, so that they can enjoy a lifetime of mobility.

Once the spine has been aligned and all structures are free from compression or impingement, then it is time to focus on core strengthening. But what does that really mean? Are all abdominal strengtheners alike? How do we access the deep, internal stabilizers while maintaining back health, especially after an injury? Can abdominal exercises create harm? These are just some of the questions I will discuss and answer in this chapter.

In her *True Refuge* (2013), psychologist Tara Brach describes a "space suit" that we often wear in order to protect the more vulnerable true self, which is at our core. Her description of this image and process is worth quoting in full:

> We are born with a beautiful open spirit, alive with innocence and resilience. But we bring this goodness into a difficult world.
>
> Imagine that at the moment of birth we begin to develop a space suit to help us navigate our strange new environment. The purpose of this space suit is to protect us from violence and greed and to win nurturance from caretakers who, to varying degrees, are bound by their own self-absorption and insecurities. When our needs aren't met, our space suit creates the best defensive and proactive strategies it can. These include tensions in the body and emotions such as anger, anxiety, and shame; mental activity such as judging, obsessing, and fantasizing; and a whole array of behavioral tactics for going after whatever is missing—security, food, sex, love.
>
> Our space suit is essential for survival, and some of its strategies do help us become productive, stable, and responsible adults. And yet the same space suit that protects us can also prevent us from moving spontaneously, joyfully, and freely through our lives.
>
> This is when our space suit becomes our prison. (p.16)

While Brach has created a powerful analogy for the human psyche and the way we operate in the world, the same analogy can be used to understand our physical bodies and, more specifically, the abdominals. Very often we are more concerned with our outward appearance than our inner resilience, and we therefore spend a great deal of time perfecting our "outer self" rather than focusing on our "inner self." When helping clients strengthen the core, I often feel that individuals are trying to build a "suit of armor" rather than integrity from the inside out. My teacher often said that if we spent as much time in meditation and self-reflection as we do on perfecting our appearance, we would be a society of very enlightened beings. Instead, for fear of appearing vulnerable or too sensitive, we spend countless hours on our "walls," only to find our foundation crumbling beneath us. When things fall apart, this is often the time when we are forced to make changes, and back pain can be one of those opportunities to start doing things differently. We may be forced to look at how we have been building walls, literally and metaphorically, in order to protect a fragile and weak inner self. The process of understanding this begins with the body, but, if the physical work is done right, we may then be able to take a closer look at something deep inside that is desperately seeking attention and healing.

Sometimes trying too hard creates more rigidity throughout the body. Your students and clients, who tend to co-contract their abdominals and back muscles intentionally during exercise, can actually cause increased compression in the spine and, as Mens *et al.* (2006) contend, can create damaging forces on pelvic ligaments. Also, by instructing clients to hold a "neutral spine," we may perpetuate the guarding, the rigid bracing, reduced movement, altered breathing pattern, and muscular inefficiency by activating more muscle groups than required. This is often the case, Prosko (2014) discovered, in individuals with back pain. They either turn everything on or everything off. As yoga therapists, our job is to teach our clients how to balance the contraction in some muscles and simultaneous relaxation in other muscles during the postures. With this in mind, it is preferable to have clients with back pain move in pain-free ranges of movement while becoming aware that they can activate the abdominals without forcing or gripping. Watch their faces. Is there tension in the eyes and the forehead? How about the jaw? Are the shoulders riding up towards the ears? Does the trunk look rigid? These are clues that they are probably holding unnecessary tension in their bodies and minds. This is a good time to recommend that they turn the corners of their lips up, as a gentle inner smile will soften all these areas. Of course, when looking at all the koshas, it is important also to get to the reason for that tension and rigidity: the source is usually core beliefs that create inner tension and pain patterns. Davis *et al.* (2002) ask an important question related to this issue:

> Maybe our patients should be encouraged to relax their trunk muscles rather than hold them rigid? In a study of the effects of psychological

stress during lifting it was found that mental processing/stress had a large impact on the spine. It resulted in a dramatic increase in spinal compression associated with increases in trunk muscle co-contraction and less controlled movements. (p.2646)

So, what is responsible for compression in the spine? Weak abdominals? Firing the wrong muscles? Timing of core activation? Or could back pain perhaps increase with mental stress rather than physical weakness? The answers are not clear, but the current evidence points to multiple biological, psychological, and social factors rather than to the reductionist view that involves a simple physical remedy—strengthening the transversus abdominis. As yoga therapists, I believe it's time we take a broader approach to the core.

If we stick with the analogy of the "suit of armor" then the muscles that give you "washboard abs" or a "six-pack" are the ones that are least beneficial to your spine, but look good on the outside. In contrast, the deeper muscles are barely visible on the outside but provide a great deal of stability from the inside out. The long-sought-after six-pack is created by a superficial abdominal muscle called the *rectus abdominis*. This muscle is an important stabilizer, but one of its primary functions is to flex the spine, thereby increasing lumbar flexion. The problem with this is that lumbar flexion is actually the one movement that is not recommended for individuals with disc bulges and herniations as it tends to increase their symptoms by putting more pressure on the exiting spinal nerves. When this is the case, then sit-ups (rectus abdominis strengtheners) would actually be contraindicated for back pain due to a pinched nerve or bulging disc.

Another interesting thing to note is that in yoga we see the abdomen from a very different point of view than the western fitness paradigm. *In yoga, our goal is a toned but soft abdomen.* We want to have full control and excursion of our diaphragm for pranayama and meditation, so that our nervous system is regulated and relaxed. "Holding in the abdominals in a hard and contracted manner can interfere with breathing and digestion, among other functions," says Judith Hanson Lasater in her 2009 book, *Yoga Body* (p.135). If you look at most of the yoga masters around, their bellies are slightly rounded or soft. Even the Buddha has a soft belly and seems quite happy with it. Does that mean we should let it all hang out? As in every other aspect of yoga, the ultimate goal is a balance between strength and flexibility. It is just that very often we overdo the strengthening aspect, especially when it comes to abdominals, rather than balance the strength with softness.

The abdomen is an area that is filled with nerves from the sympathetic chain. In fact, we are learning more and more that this area, called the *enteric nervous system*, is just as intuitive and intelligent as the central nervous system (CNS), and that there is a great deal of truth to having a "gut instinct" about something. In addition, our friend from Chapter 4, the psoas major, sits in the abdominal cavity and attaches directly to the diaphragm and the bodies and discs of the T12–L5 vertebrae. The psoas is one of the primary muscles that responds to stress and also has a direct impact on the lower back. It is with this in mind that I consider this muscle a large part of our "core."

What is the core exactly?

Before we dive into the anatomy of the core, I would encourage you to ask your clients, "What does the core mean to you on an energetic level?" Then have them ask themselves a series of questions such as these:

- "What is at your core?"

- "What drives you?"

- "What are your core beliefs?"

- "What is deep inside that you hold central, perhaps something that no one else is allowed or able to see from the outside?"

- "Is there somewhere in your being that you are not acting in accordance with your integrity?"

To me, these questions are just as important, if not more so, than examining whether the transversus abdominis and multifidus are firing in plank pose or not.

You see, at our core, we can see where our weaknesses lie. We can see where we feel scared and alone, unsupported, and out of control. If we tune in to those emotions, we can also learn how to soften the muscles that need to relax—namely, the psoas, the erector spinae group, the quadratus lumborum, the upper trapezius, and especially the diaphragm. We can also learn how to be strong without having to "be tight and hard" or "having to hold our breath in." *This is what true core strength is.* It all comes back to one of the few *Yoga Sutras of Patanjali* (see Satchidananda 1978/2010) that refer to the physical practice of yoga asana (postures): *sthira-sukham-asanam*. This wisdom means balancing steadiness and sweetness, or strength and comfort, in yoga poses. It is further defined on the Ashtanga Yoga website's source-texts page: "practicing yoga with strength and in a relaxed manner gives rise to harmony with the physical body (asana)" (p.2, verse 42). This balance of steadiness and relaxation was taught hundreds of years ago in the *Yoga Sutras of Patanjali*, but continues to hold true to this day. We need to know when to stand our ground and when to let go. We need to teach our students how to be strong and soft at the same time. This effort to find balance, the right combination of softness and strength, is the main difference between yoga therapy and other forms of physical exercise and rehabilitation.

A dear colleague of mine, Shelly Prosko, explains that core work is "less about core strength or stability" than it is about what she calls "core timing." We want to be sensitive to when our muscles are firing in order to provide support during functional activities. Sensitivity can only occur when we bring awareness and breath into the movement, which, in turn, means slowing down and paying attention. It is because of this that, in my mentorship program, I have my students focus on "slowing down" their practice in the first month of training. I do not particularly care what asana they choose to practice, as long as it is done slowly. If we are moving quickly from pose to pose with loud music in the background, how can we tune in to our bodies' subtle activities?

Anatomy of the core

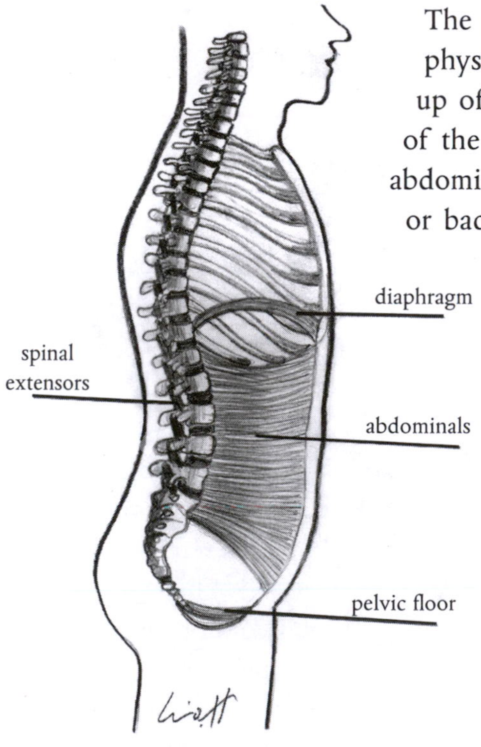

Figure 7.1 The core

The generally accepted understanding of the physical core of the body is that it is made up of many muscles that support the integrity of the trunk. Anteriorly, the body has the four abdominal muscles; posteriorly, the spinal muscles or back extensors; inferiorly, there is the pelvic floor; and superiorly, the diaphragm. These muscles form a cylinder that supports the spine and pelvis.

In addition, there are other muscles that can be considered a part of the core, including the psoas major and iliacus, quadratus lumborum, and latissimus dorsi, as well as the many muscles that control scapular stability. First let's explore the abdominals from superficial to deep; these muscles comprise the anterior wall of the core.

1. Rectus abdominis

This paired muscle runs vertically down the abdominal region and originates on the crest of the pubis and pubic symphysis. It then attaches to the xiphoid process and the costal cartilage of ribs V–VII. It is separated by the linea alba, a band of connective tissue down the center, as well as multiple horizontal bands of tendinous tissue which creates the look of the six- or eight-pack. Its function is trunk flexion and stabilization. It can also help in forced exhalation.

2. External obliques

Starting from the inferior border of the lower eight ribs, these muscles go in a diagonal direction and insert into the anterior portions of the iliac crests, as well as into the linea alba. Their main action is twisting, combined with the internal obliques, but can also help to flex the trunk and aid in forced exhalation.

3. Internal obliques

The fibers of the internal obliques go in the opposite direction to the external obliques. They originate from the thoraco-lumbar fascia, inguinal ligament, and lateral iliac crest, and insert into the linea alba and the inferior borders of ribs X–XII.

4. Transversus abdominis (TA)

The TA has developed some notoriety in the world of core strengthening as the most important muscle to target for increased spinal stability. This is largely based on one study (1996) by Hodges and Richardson that found a delay in the firing of the TA and multifidus muscles in individuals with lower back pain.

The TA behaves like an internal corset or brace placed horizontally across the abdomen from the lateral inguinal ligament, anterior iliac crests, and thoraco-lumbar fascia; it then inserts into the linea alba. When it contracts it provides stability by compressing the abdominal contents. It also plays a part in forced exhalation.

In "The myth of core stability" Lederman (2007) questions the significance of the findings of Hodges and his collaborators. He doubts the effect of the delay in firing of the TA and argues that most individuals with back pain will have altered firing patterns of muscles anyway, so, in truth, it is a question of the chicken and the egg (p.12). Is this enough proof that TA strengthening will actually relieve back pain and increase stability when isolated? Or is the TA just one of many trunk stabilizers that need to be worked functionally for optimal performance and pain reduction?

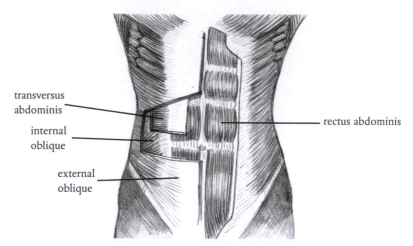

Figure 7.2 The four abdominal muscles

The posterior wall of the core is made up of a number of back muscles, including the erector spinae group, quadratus lumborum, latissimus dorsi, trapezius, and serratus anterior. All these muscles need to work with proper timing and sequencing to support the spine during functional activities and during asana alike. For our purposes, we will focus mostly on the deep spinal muscle, the multifidus, which is the one responsible for spinal stability and also has been shown to have a direct connection with the transversus abdominis. But it is important to remember that all trunk muscles work together to create spinal stability that is best trained through functional activities.

5. Multifidus

This muscle consists of smaller muscles that provide spinal stability as they connect the vertebrae to one another alongside the spine. The muscle runs from the sacrum (posterior iliac spine and posterior sacroiliac ligaments) and from the mamillary and transverse processes to the spinous processes of the vertebrae above, in a superomedial direction.

Research shows a direct connection between the ability to fire the multifidus muscle and TA activation. There is a 4.5× increase in the likelihood of contraction of these deep spinal muscles when the TA is accessed. In addition, Hides *et al.* (2011) have shown that there is an association between weakness in the multifidus on one side and unilateral back pain in the same area. Researchers have concluded that it is helpful to work on contracting these spinal stabilizers when working with individuals with lower back pain.

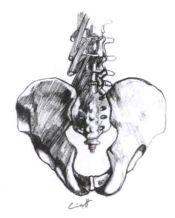

Figure 7.3 The multifidus (deep spinal extensors)

The roof of the core is made up of the diaphragm, which is a dome-shaped muscle that inserts into itself at a common tendon. Because the diaphragm is such a clear part of the core of the body, it should be obvious that focusing on proper breathing must be an integral part of rehabilitation for back pain.

6. The diaphragm

This thin band of skeletal muscle separates the thoracic cavity from the abdominal cavity. It originates anteriorly on the xiphoid process and costal margins, laterally on ribs VI–XII and posteriorly on T12. There is also an attachment via the left and right crus (tendon-like structures) to the lumbar vertebrae at L1–L2. As previously stated, the muscle inserts into its own central tendon, and when it contracts, it creates negative pressure in the thoracic cavity, so that air can be drawn into the lungs for respiration. Expiration is a function of the passive recoiling of the diaphragm back to its original position. Forced exhalation requires muscular activation of abdominal muscles and intercostals.

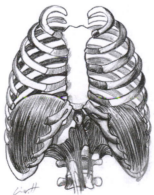

Figure 7.4 The diaphragm

The importance of working with the diaphragm to achieve proper breathing cannot be emphasized enough when working from the perspective of yoga therapy. On a physical level, proper diaphragmatic excursion helps increase trunk mobility, as the diaphragm is directly connected to the rib cage and thoracic spine. In fact, in my practice I have noticed that most individuals who have lower back pain have decreased mobility in the thoracic spine. This, in turn, creates too much mobility in the already weakened lumbar spine.

We have to train ourselves always to look at areas of the body as parts of the larger and more integrated kinetic chain. Increased strain on the lumbar spine usually occurs because other systems in the chain are not taking up their workload. If there is decreased trunk mobility, decreased rib excursion during breathing, increased accessory muscle use, tight hip musculature, or pelvic imbalance, each of these factors can contribute to increased loading on the lower back. By addressing only the physical structures in the lower back, we are missing the point. We want to look for the source of the problem and help our clients and students find more balance, so that there is healthy loading of the spine throughout the natural curves. This lack of balance is often why surgery does not provide an adequate solution to the problem. Even if the disc is removed or the spine is fused, the loading will still be out of balance if the structures above and below the injury are not dealt with.

Proper breathing also has the most significant effect on the nervous system, which is the key to relaxing the deep muscles that tighten and contribute to spinal compression. In addition, the breath directly affects your students' emotional landscape, and vice versa. Emotions such as fear and anxiety, as well as lack of control and lack of trust, will cause shallow, short breaths that increase neck and back tension and shift the nervous system into the sympathetic fight-or-flight mode. In addition to the added muscular tension, the body's ability to send oxygen and nutrients to the muscles and joints in order to repair itself is impaired in this state.

When in doubt, work on the breath! It is the most important component, as it encompasses all five koshas in an accessible way and will help your students and clients achieve both physical and emotional well-being.

7. The pelvic floor

Finally, the infamous and mysterious pelvic floor makes up the bottom layer of the "core." It is considered a diaphragm just like the one above, and is also called the *urogenital diaphragm*.

The pelvic floor consists of the levator ani muscle, the coccygeus, and connective tissue, that make up the bottom of the pelvic cavity. The levator ani is usually considered in three parts: pubococcygeus, puborectalis, and iliococcygeus. This structure is important for support of the pelvic organs, including the bladder, intestines and uterus. It also plays an important role in continence and childbirth. Most people are not aware of their pelvic floor until something goes wrong in that area.

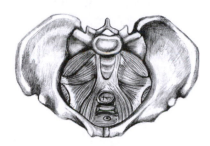

Figure 7.5 The pelvic floor

When most people think about pelvic floor dysfunction, they think about weakness and overstretched muscles. These are a few of the problems that can contribute to urgency, incontinence, and pain. There is, however, another, less obvious form of pelvic floor dysfunction that can lead to pain and incontinence as well: hypertonicity. Hypertonicity, as described by Sapsford (2004), refers to over-contraction and spasm of the pelvic floor muscles, where constant gripping causes fatigue in the muscles, which then leads to incontinence. So, just as in the abdominals, there can be too much tension held in the pelvic floor, contributing to incontinence as well. Kumar, Kumar, and Kumar (2012) have also shown that there is a direct correlation between pelvic floor dysfunction, lower back pain, and sacroiliac joint dysfunction (pp. 1–3).

In "Rehabilitation of pelvic floor muscles utilizing trunk stabilization," Sapsford (2004) also points to a much discussed theory in the yoga and research community that sees a connection of posture to the psoas and transversus abdominis, which share a common fascial sheath with the pelvic floor. Both the diaphragm and the TA should expand gently with the inhalation and contract with the exhalation. In the event of a poor sitting posture, the chest is collapsed while the psoas hip flexor is tight and pulls on this fascial sheath; this affects how the diaphragm and TA can expand and contract. The result is shorter breath and less support for the pelvic floor region, since the abs are unable to contract efficiently. McLean (2015) notes that when the abdominals can contract efficiently they assist the pelvic floor muscles in controlling the pelvic floor region.

Proper alignment of the pelvis will also affect your client's ability to control the activation of the pelvic floor muscles. If the pelvis is tipped backwards in a posterior tilt, common to the faulty position many of us adopt when sitting in a chair, it is very difficult to effectively contract the pelvic floor musculature. When your student or client begins to bring the pelvis into more of an anterior tilt, which in turn restores the natural lumbar curve, proper activation of these muscles is optimized. In conclusion, the pelvic floor muscles can be either too tight or too weak, and are directly affected by the position of the spine and pelvic bowl. Based on this information, we can conclude that spine health is directly related to healthy pelvic floor activation.

PRACTICE TIP 13

Try tucking the tailbone and firing the pelvic floor at the same time:

- Sit on the floor or on a pillow and begin to move the pelvis into an anterior and posterior pelvic tilt. As you do that, pay attention to your ability to feel and access your pelvic floor.

- Next, round your shoulders and slouch, placing the pelvis in a posterior tilt. While in this position, try to lift and engage the pelvic floor muscles. Notice your ability to fire them as well as the strength of your contraction.

- Now tilt the pelvis anteriorly and find a natural lumbar curve. In this position, begin to contract the pelvic floor muscles and notice if there is a difference in your ability to activate them and the strength of the contraction.

- Observe and feel the relationship between the pelvis and the ease of activation of your pelvic floor. What do you find regarding the connection of your posture and your ability to activate this area?

Connecting to the core

Based on this discussion, your clients and students will build a stable center from which to move, not so much by becoming stronger in the core but rather by knowing how to connect to the muscles of the core. If we make the exercises harder, but are not accessing the right muscles, we could actually be making the problem worse and putting more strain on the lower back area.

One of the more common muscles that will fire to compensate for weak abdominals is psoas major. When the abdominals are weak, these powerful hip flexors contract to bring the torso towards the thigh and vice versa. Very often in yoga, we can find crafty ways to avoid accessing the deep spinal stabilizers, and more often than not, this is a function of the ego wanting to push beyond our true physical limitations.

A perfect example of this avoidance and pushing can be seen in the yoga posture called boat pose or Navasana, one of the common abdominal strengtheners taught in class. While Navasana *is* an abdominal strengthener, we tend to use our hip flexors in order to keep the legs elevated in the pose. When we straighten our legs, more force is required to hold the weight of the legs in the air; this creates a burning sensation in the frontal hip creases. This effect is exacerbated for individuals who have a shorter torso and longer legs (see Figure 7.6 a.), something I noticed a few years ago in my own personal practice. For those with a longer torso and shorter legs, the weight is more evenly distributed, the core is more easily accessed, and it is easier to hold the legs aloft (see Figure 7.6 b.). Very often, those of us blessed with long legs experience increased stress on the lumbar spine and hip flexors in this pose. As a guideline, have your students straighten their legs only to the point where the toes are at the level of their forehead. That will help them access the core more efficiently and avoid overengaging the psoas. You might also instruct your students or clients to try the next practice tip.

a.   b.

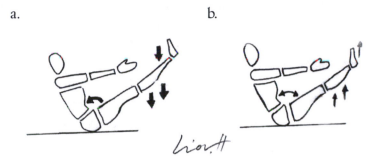

Figure 7.6 Load on the psoas in: a. individuals with longer legs and shorter torso; b. those with shorter legs and longer torso

PRACTICE TIP 14

Practice Navasana and experiment with bending the knees vs. straightening the legs. Notice where you feel the work. Hold for a little longer and notice if there is a feeling of tension or tightening in the hip flexors. If you feel the work in the anterior hip area, start bending your knees only to the point where you feel the work in the abdominal area. That is the place where you should work for a while. Continue to work here and practice longer holds before straightening your legs any further. Begin to be aware of the messages your mind is sending to you. Notice the tendency to want to go further even though you know that you may not be accessing the correct muscles. Where is that drive coming from? Is there a message or voice that you are hearing, telling you that you are not good enough? That you are not working hard enough? That you could do better?

Acknowledge that voice and kindly give yourself permission to practice this posture with awareness of your core. Give yourself permission not to push toward your edge but rather to listen to what would benefit you most today. Even if slightly uncomfortable, smile from a place deep inside, knowing that you are being a little kinder to yourself today and decreasing the load on your spine.

There is yet another detail that is important for your students or clients to observe in Navasana. Yoga teachers still discuss and often disagree about the correct position of the lumbar spine in boat pose. Some instructors prefer an arch in the lower back in this pose, while others recommend slight lumbar flexion. I encourage you to ask your students or clients to practice and feel both versions in their bodies. Then ask them what they notice.

As always in yoga, I believe we all need to find a delicate balance between the two possibilities. As Judith Hanson Lasater (2009) writes in *Yoga Body*, "It is important to the health of the lumbar spine, in order to maintain the integrity of the pose, that you remain in (lumbar) flexion, using the strength of your abdominals and hip flexors. Do not lift your chest; this extends the lumbar spine and puts the abdominals at a mechanical disadvantage" (p. 140). If there is too much extension in the lumbar spine, the iliopsoas will fire more than the abdominal muscles, since their action is to create extension in the lumbar spine when engaged bilaterally. Conversely, if the lumbar spine is set up in a slightly flexed position, the rectus abdominis is at a mechanical advantage to fire over the more powerful hip flexors and can be engaged more readily. This does not mean, however, that we want the shoulders to round forward. The idea is to shift the weight slightly back onto the base of the sacrum, so that the lower lumbar spine is in gentle flexion, while lifting the sternum and encouraging slight extension in the thoracic spine, so that the chest stays open throughout the pose. This is the dance of Navasana.

Here is the way to instruct students or clients with back pain to progress in boat pose:

1. Start in a seated position with knees bent and feet on the floor. Hold behind the knees and lean backwards, rounding the abdomen slightly so that you feel your abdominal muscles working.

2. Next, slowly lift one leg so that your shinbone is parallel to the floor. Hold there for a few breaths, feeling the work in the lower belly area. Then place the foot on the ground and repeat by lifting the other leg. If there is any pain in the lower back or if you feel your hip flexors working more than the abdominals, back off and keep both feet on the floor.

3. To progress, lift both legs off the ground while holding onto the backs of the knees. Draw the belly button towards the spine on each exhalation, as you maintain lumbar flexion throughout the pose. Start to extend the time spent in the posture.

4. The next step is to extend your arms out to the side while keeping the knees bent. Keep your knees close together, as if you are squeezing a ball between your inner thighs. Start to focus on the relationship between the inner thighs, pelvic floor, and abdominals.

5. The final pose is done with straight legs and arms extended alongside the body, as long as you feel the work in the abdominal area. Play with straightening your knees and bending them, finding the right posture for your body so that you can maintain the integrity of the pose. Watch your ego here, for it is bound to get in the way. Smile at your ego and do what is best for you at this moment.

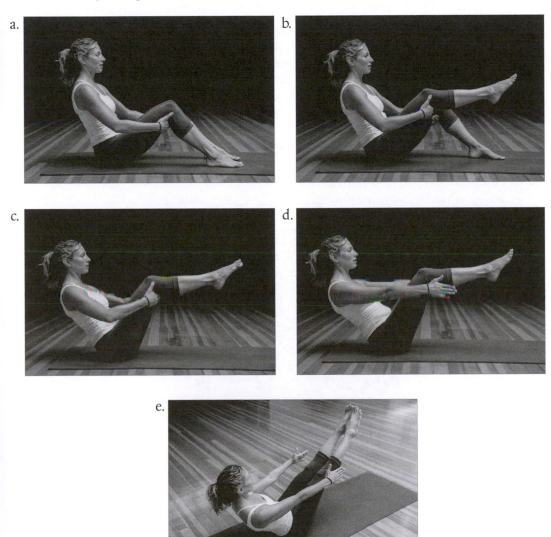

Figure 7.7 a. Navasana with both feet on ground; b. one leg lifted; c. both legs lifted, knees bent; d. arms extended and knees bent; e. with legs extended

While most individuals enjoy the sensation of "burning" in their hip joints and thighs, I believe that most people wrongly focus on strengthening their hip flexors, which are already in a state of tension and contribute to increased spinal compression. Instead, as Liz Koch (1981/2012) writes in *The Psoas Book*, "People do not have 'weak' psoas muscles that need strengthening through standard muscle protocols; they have exhausted psoas muscles often due to an overwhelmed nervous system. The exhausted muscle is only thought to be weak because it behaves unresponsively" (p.44). Most people really need to focus more on releasing tension in the psoas, rather than strengthening it and contributing to increased tightness and, consequently, increased pressure on the lumbar spine.

It is for this reason that I do not teach poses such as Utthita Hasta Padangusthasana (standing hand to big toe pose) in my Happy Back yoga classes (see Figure 7.8). This pose requires a great deal of work in the hip flexors to hold the extended leg out against gravity, thereby contributing to increased pressure on the lower back by tensing the psoas and rectus femoris muscles. Why work on this pose when there are many other postures that do not carry the risk of stressing the hip flexors and lower back? I feel that when you are teaching students in a Happy Back yoga class, it is more beneficial to work on postures that strengthen the core while simultaneously encouraging a release in the psoas and other hip flexors.

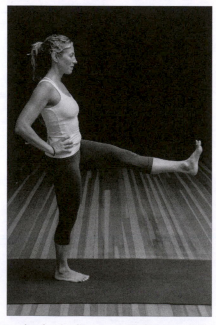

Figure 7.8 Standing hand to big toe pose (Utthita Hasta Padangusthasana)

Below is a series of abdominal strengtheners that I recommend to include in your yoga classes and private sessions for individuals with back pain.

1. Lifting the pit of the abdomen

Begin working with clients by having them lie on their backs with the knees bent and feet on the floor. The reason it is helpful to start in a supine position is that it is much easier to access the pit of the abdomen (POA) here than in standing, especially during the postures that require more intricate balance and awareness. By taking gravity out of the equation, your students will succeed in bringing more awareness to this area that is often forgotten or inaccessible.

I recommend that you begin with the technique described in Chapter 3, finding the POA with a stick. The POA is the area between the navel and the pubic bone and is comprised of the transversus abdominis, rectus abdominis, and external and internal obliques.

To find it, have your student lie on her back and place her hands on her belly below the navel. Invite her to take a deep inhalation and feel the belly rise, and then exhale, feeling the belly fall under her hands. *On the next exhalation, ask her to draw the lower belly area back towards the spine and up toward the head.* Repeat this action with each exhalation, relaxing the belly on the inhalation. Then have the student place a long stick in the area just beneath the navel and above the pubic bone. She should feel the gentle pressure of the stick on the lower belly as it gives direct feedback to this area. One end of the stick should be resting against a wall. On the next exhalation, have the student lift the POA and observe the stick as it slides down the wall. Every time she draws the belly back towards the spine and up towards the head, the stick should slide down the wall. The student will be able to retrain this area with the help of this prop. Once the student can consistently move the stick by controlling the POA, she can practice without the stick in supine, then in standing, and then during yoga poses.

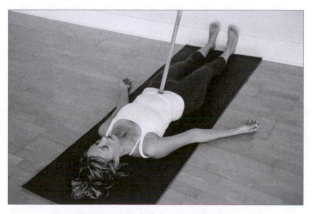

Figure 7.9 Rod placement in the POA

2. Arm lift on all fours

Have your students come onto all fours by placing their hands under their shoulder joints and knees directly underneath the hips. The lumbar spine should be in a perfectly neutral position, which means that there should be a natural small arch in the lower back. On the next exhalation, have them draw the navel towards the spine and lift one arm up to the level of the ear, or above. Have them hold the arm out until they feel significant work in the abdominal area. Hold here for 30 seconds to one minute and switch sides. This is an excellent pose to access the abdominals for individuals who have neck pain and have a hard time in poses that require lifting the head off the ground against gravity, since in this pose the neck remains in a neutral position.

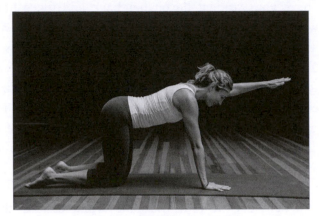

Figure 7.10 Lifting the arm on all fours

3. Supine leg lift

Another simple but effective pose that I learned from Judith Hanson Lasater is listed on page 35 of her book *Yoga Abs* (2005). This posture requires using the abdominals as stabilizers instead of as prime movers. The student begins the exercise lying supine with legs extended. On the exhalation, have her draw the belly button towards the spine and press the lower back into the ground as she lifts one leg five or so inches off the ground. The emphasis should be on feeling the abdominals stabilize the trunk while the leg is suspended for a few seconds. Then lower the leg and repeat on the other side.

To make this more challenging, the student can lift the leg up and then move the extended leg out to the side approximately ten inches. Moving the leg off to the side encourages the abdominals to stabilize the trunk even more, so that the weight of the leg doesn't pull the trunk into rotation. Hold for five seconds here, and then take the leg up a few inches and out to the side again. Take the leg up and out one more time for a total of three repetitions, and then bring the leg back to center and lower it down slowly, with control.

Note: The lower back should maintain full contact with the floor for the duration of this exercise.

a. 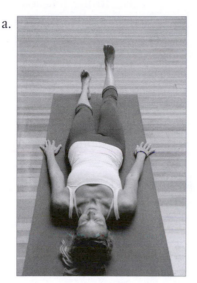   b.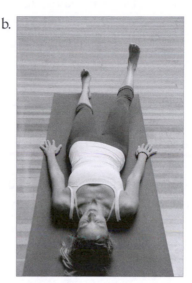

Figure 7.11 Supine leg lifts: a. straight up; b. out to the side

4. Jathara Parivartanasana/revolved abdomen pose

This is one of my favorite postures, as it encourages activation of the obliques as well as all the spinal stabilizers. The full posture can put strain on the lower back if the practitioner is not strong enough to stabilize the trunk with the core as it is traditionally practiced, with extended legs. For back health, I prefer to teach this pose with the knees bent and legs squeezing in towards one another. This puts less strain on the lower back and enables the student to pay attention to the alignment principle of keeping the knees stacked; it also gives them the ability to access the abdominals with more awareness and precision.

Have your student lie on her back with the arms extended out at shoulder height, palms facing upward. Instruct her to keep the shoulders pressing into the ground in order to maintain stability in the trunk while the legs move from side to side. Have her inhale with both legs at a 90° angle in the center. On the exhalation, instruct your client to bring the knees to the right, keeping one knee stacked directly on top of the other. (The tendency in this pose is for the top leg to slide backwards. Instead keep the pelvis moving as one unit; this requires increased awareness to keep the knees in line.) Tell your student that she should feel the work in her abdominal area, and to take the legs as far as she can only while maintaining most of the work in the core (hence avoiding lower back strain, or other muscles taking over). Hold here for one breath, and on the next exhalation have the student press her left shoulder into the ground and move the belly button and lower belly towards the left shoulder in a diagonal direction. Once in the center, take another inhalation, and on the exhalation move the legs, knees stacked, to the left, keeping the right shoulder glued to the earth. Take one deep breath here, stabilizing with the abdominal muscles. Then on the next exhalation she should draw the navel towards the right shoulder as she brings her legs back to the center using the core.

Repeat ten times to each side, alternating sides. Increase repetitions as tolerated. It is also recommended to lower the legs more towards the ground as the student gets stronger, to increase the load on the abdominals and spinal stabilizers.

The full posture is practiced with the legs extended and moving up towards the opposite shoulder. This is an advanced variation of the pose and should only be practiced by students who can effectively use their abdominals instead of their back muscles.

a. 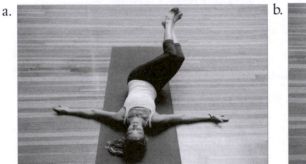 b.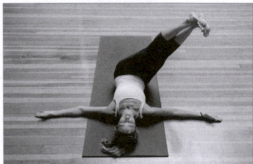

Figure 7.12 Jathara Parivartanasana: a. with knees bent (preferred for back issues); b. with legs straight

5. Phalakasana/plank pose

This remains one of the best ways to strengthen the core, as it does a great job of encouraging the core to do its work as a trunk stabilizer and teaches the deeper muscles to protect the lumbar spine. In addition, it is an excellent strengthener for the serratus anterior muscles, which help to stabilize the shoulder blades and release neck tension. Plank pose can be practiced either with the arms extended or on the forearms, which may be easier for individuals with wrist pain. Have your students practice this pose with the knees on the ground first, before extending the legs, to make sure they are strong enough to maintain a natural curve in the lower back throughout the duration of the posture. In order to feel the work in the abdominal area, it is important to come into full plank and then drop the knees to the ground so that they are positioned correctly.

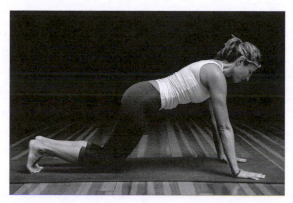

Figure 7.13 Correct positioning of knees in modified plank pose

If your student can maintain the integrity of the lumbar spine in this pose with the knees off the ground, then she can practice the next variation. With extended arms, have her press all finger mounds firmly into the ground, spreading the shoulder blades and filling up the space between the shoulder blades. (In other words, instruct her not to allow the shoulder blades to come towards one another, which will create a "valley" between the shoulder blades.) On the exhalation, make sure your student is drawing the navel towards the spine and keeping the legs very active and energized, squeezing them together firmly.

If your client is performing the pose on forearms, make sure the elbows stay in line with the shoulders, and that she presses the entire length of the forearms into the ground. Have her work on increasing her time in this pose from 30 to 90 seconds.

Shaking is normal in this posture; however, if there is sinking in the lower back, the student is not strong enough to hold the pose and needs to rest. Eventually, with practice, she will begin to hold longer and with more integrity.

a.

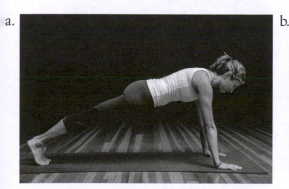

b.

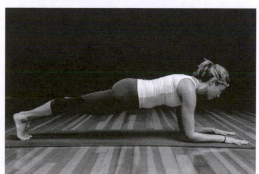

Figure 7.14 a. Plank (Phalakasana) on extended arms; b. plank on forearms

6. Vasisthasana/side plank

The full pose is practiced on an extended arm while raising the pelvis away from the ground, thereby contracting the side of the body by moving the pelvic rim towards the lower ribs. This requires a great deal of strength in the arm as well as the trunk. In addition, this one pose was shown in a research article by Fishman, Groessl, and Sherman (2014) to help improve scoliosis in individuals when practiced for 90 seconds a day on the convex side of the curve. In fact, the study concluded that an average of 32 percent improvement was noted in the curves of individuals who remained committed to the protocol. The philosophy of this protocol is to strengthen the muscles that are lengthened and weakened by the pull of the tighter muscles on the concave side of the curve.

Because of the difficulty of the posture, including pressure on the wrists, a few variations may be helpful to begin with. See Figure 7.15 for different variations that you can use to make this pose accessible to your students and/ or clients.

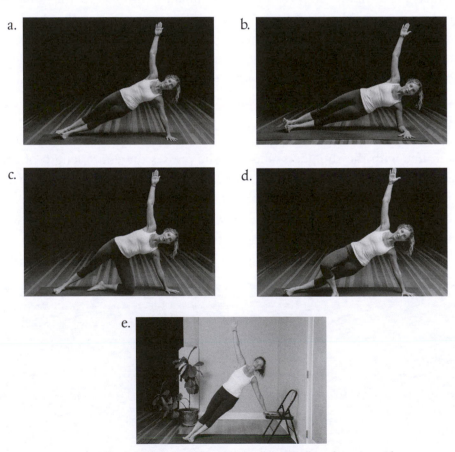

Figure 7.15 Side plank (Vasisthasana): a. traditional variation; b. on forearm; c. with one knee on the ground; d. with top leg crossed over the bottom leg; e. using a chair

What I have noticed in my practice and from working with individuals with lower back pain is that the best treatment does not necessarily involve coming up with harder or more creative abdominal exercises, but rather with helping them learn how to access the core in a few well-designed, well-practiced postures with lots of mindfulness. Doing this takes a great deal of honesty and self-awareness on the part of the practitioner. In looking at myself and even at other individuals when they are practicing yoga, I have seen that working the core is a good way to begin to face your ego head on.

The ego will want to make it harder in order to prove that it can maintain the position at all costs. Notice if your client falls into this category. Ask him or her to be honest and to ask: "Who are you really kidding?" Explain that when you take yourself beyond your limits, all you end up doing is hurting yourself and making your back pain worse. Somehow, even knowing this, you may notice your students pushing themselves beyond their abilities. Encourage them to take the pose down a notch and choose an easier variation than the one they immediately jumped to. See if they can hold this "easier posture" for 60 to 90 seconds while maintaining perfect integrity in the trunk and pelvis. Encourage them to breathe and to find the place in the pose where there is steadiness and comfort (*sthira-sukham-asanam*), where they can be strong and relaxed at the same time, without unnecessarily making the spinal muscles hard and tense.

We all want to do the more advanced variation of the pose, but if we go too far, we impact the lower back and don't strengthen the abdominals at all. Here are a few tips to help your clients get the most out of their core:

1. *Keep it simple and consistent.* Practice the above exercises and maintain consistency, rather than trying many new abdominal exercises that run the risk of increasing tension in the hip flexors. Once again, it comes back to awareness. Have your students and clients ask themselves, "Am I really accessing the right muscles?" Have them notice if their mind is telling them they need to progress faster than they are able. Create a safe place for them to remain aware and feel what is happening in their body as they try the different variations of the pose.

2. *Maintain the natural curves of the spine.* If posture is off, the diaphragm isn't able to work efficiently. In addition, the pelvic floor and abdominal muscles are compromised when the spine and pelvis are out of alignment.

3. *Focus on inner strength.* Core work is less about achieving washboard abs and more about finding deeper strength. Create the intention of focusing on your inner resilience and integrity in your practice.

4. *Keep perspective.* As in yoga, core stability is less about the shape of your body and more about the shape of your life. Your goal is not to show off or to have the flattest abs in town, but rather to know what is best for you at any given moment; to have enough strength balanced with softness and vulnerability, so that you can shed that "space suit" and live more fully from your heart each day and with each interaction.

5. *Rest in your integrity.* Find the place where you can hold the pose and feel the abdominals for a while. If you lose strength easily there, choose a slightly less strenuous modification. Progress by lengthening the time spent in each pose instead of taking it too far, too fast.

What is core stability really about in yoga therapy?

Core strength is not about building outer walls or having "strong abdominals" but is rather about building inner resilience and balancing strength with softness and an air of surrender.

It is about being in your integrity, knowing who you are and standing strong in the face of others doubting you. In *Fire of Love*, my teacher Aadil Palkhivala (2008a) quotes a poem by Rudyard Kipling (1865–1936) that I have never forgotten since we read it aloud in teacher training. I believe that this poem represents what we strive for in yoga and in life.

If

IF you can keep your head when all about you
Are losing theirs and blaming it on you,
If you can trust yourself when all men doubt you,
But make allowance for their doubting too;
If you can wait and not be tired by waiting,
Or being lied about, don't deal in lies,
Or being hated, don't give way to hating,
And yet don't look too good, nor talk too wise:

If you can dream—and not make dreams your master;
If you can think—and not make thoughts your aim;

If you can meet with Triumph and Disaster

And treat those two impostors just the same;

If you can bear to hear the truth you've spoken

Twisted by knaves to make a trap for fools,

Or watch the things you gave your life to, broken,

And stoop and build 'em up with worn-out tools:

If you can make one heap of all your winnings

And risk it on one turn of pitch-and-toss,

And lose, and start again at your beginnings

And never breathe a word about your loss;

If you can force your heart and nerve and sinew

To serve your turn long after they are gone,

And so hold on when there is nothing in you

Except the Will which says to them: "Hold on!"

If you can talk with crowds and keep your virtue,

Or walk with Kings—nor lose the common touch,

If neither foes nor loving friends can hurt you,

If all men count with you, but none too much;

If you can fill the unforgiving minute

With sixty seconds' worth of distance run,

Yours is the Earth and everything that's in it,

And—which is more—you'll be a Man, my son!

Yoga is as much about restraint as it is about opening. We want our students to open their chests, but without dumping into their lower backs in the process. We want them to activate the pit of the abdomen in poses like Virabhadrasana I/warrior I and Ustrasana/camel so that they maintain integrity and length in their spine as they move into back bends. I have noticed the tendency of some styles of yoga to turn all standing poses into back bends, as if going further is "more advanced" or "better" in some way. It is my belief that very often less is more. As a teacher or therapist it is important to watch the ego and notice where your student's desire to push farther comes from. Is it a desire to lengthen and to grow? Or is it a constant sense of "striving" or "being good enough" that is motivating them? The process of yoga therapy and healing is individualized, and therefore must be adapted so you can help balance each individual's tendencies. Some students may need to work on gaining strength, while others need more surrender. This is the true art of core strengthening. And very often, letting go is the hardest part of it all.

CASE STUDY: MARK

Treatment Session 5

Mark falls into the "all or nothing" category mentioned earlier in this chapter. Instead of seeing weakness in his abdominal area, my assessment of him is that he is too rigid and guarded. He has learned, over the years, to "maintain a stiff upper lip" and never to show that he is weak in any way. Consequently he has learned to contract all his muscles at the same time in order to produce a sturdy and bullet-proof "space suit." Yes, his abdominal muscles are strong, but they are also hard and inflexible, as are his back extensors, neck muscles, and psoas major. His breathing is short and shallow and his diaphragm excursion is limited, decreasing mobility in his thoracic spine and rib cage. In addition, he tends to stand in a posterior pelvic tilt, putting the pelvic floor musculature at a disadvantage. He seems to be "holding on for dear life" by maintaining tightness throughout his body and especially in his forehead and jaw.

For someone like Mark we need to emphasize the aspect of letting go and becoming more soft and flexible in the core.

We began the session by coming back to Tadasana and finding the natural curves in the spine so that he could access his pelvic floor. Then, in Tadasana, we worked on focused breathing into his diaphragm and pelvic floor. As he inhaled, he imagined the diaphragm descending and the abdominal contents being pushed forward. I encouraged him to let his belly puff out on the inhalation, as that is what it is supposed to do biomechanically. We then moved on to feeling the inhalation and its effect on the pelvic floor and its descent.

On the exhalation, Mark focused on lifting the pit of the abdomen (POA) while maintaining the natural curves of the spine. At the same time, he focused on a gentle lift of the pelvic floor. Throughout this process he was reminded to relax his face and neck muscles. I would sometimes coax him to smile or laugh so that he would let go of some of the oppressive tension that I could see in his forehead. I encouraged him to have fun with this exercise and not to take it so seriously. I taught him that it is possible to have effort and ease during the same posture, and how to separate the muscles that should be active from those that should remain relaxed and at rest.

Afterwards we worked on some gentle abdominal strengtheners, again with the emphasis being on feeling the work in the front of the body and keeping the hip flexors and back extensors soft and supple. I chose to teach him plank pose on extended arms and Jathara Parivartanasana (revolved abdomen pose) so that he worked on overall stabilization in neutral and with recruitment of the obliques as well. I emphasized the need to slow down and feel what is happening. Instead of working at his maximum capacity, I had him practice the exercises with effort at about 70 percent of where he would normally go.

In addition, we talked a lot about what feelings come up when he allows himself to soften a bit, or even when he allows himself to slow down and do less. He noticed an angry, critical voice telling him that he is "not good enough" and needs to be a "real man." He hears this voice telling him that showing any feelings or expressing any needs is a sign of weakness, and that being weak is bad.

We talk about the fact that perhaps, due to these beliefs, he has been holding so much inner tension to keep the appearance of being strong, even when he feels tired or worn out. He kept piling on more work and doing favors for other people while his personal health and energy level were dropping steadily. This created even more tension as he became quietly resentful of his boss, co-workers, and even his wife, for making too many demands on him. Mark admitted not even realizing how angry he was until we brought these things to light.

Mark left that day feeling lighter and freer than ever. Someone had seen his pain and the world did not come crashing down. His homework was to practice these three exercises, with the focus on letting go of gripping and tension while feeling a strong activation in his abdominal muscles. He was also to journal about his core beliefs and which of those might be preventing his ability to heal from his back injury.

To review, the postures prescribed were:
- Tadasana, with an emphasis on pelvic alignment and diaphragmatic and pelvic breathing
- plank pose on extended arms, with an emphasis on serratus anterior and abdominal stabilization and relaxing the upper trapezius

- Jathara Parivartanasana, only going 50-70 percent of his max and using the breath to encourage more activation of the core as he moves his legs side to side slowly.

CHAPTER 8

Getting to the Heart of the Matter

Looking Inward

**Look at the way your mind is controlling you
and it will inspire you to change.**

Prasad Ragnekar

The more I work with patients from all over the world, the more I see how clearly our outer bodies mirror our emotional and spiritual bodies. It has also become equally clear to me that unless we take a long, hard, and honest look at our beliefs and emotional landscapes, complete healing from pain will elude us.

The most obvious example that I can offer my clients who doubt the connection between musculoskeletal pain and inner tension is the relationship of emotions to the stomach. I ask them if they have ever been nervous and had butterflies in their stomach before a big test, presentation, or public speaking. Most individuals can relate to feeling physical symptoms in response to being nervous or anxious before an important event. If tension can cause a stomach ache, or difficulty eating, digesting, and/or eliminating, why wouldn't emotional stress have an effect on the muscles and tissues?

Ask your clients if they have ever felt nervous and suddenly developed pain in their upper back and shoulder blade area. Explain to them that when we become tense on the inside, our muscles respond in kind. Sometimes the muscles that tighten up are so deep in the body that we actually do not feel them tensing. Common muscles that respond directly to emotional stress, especially fear, are the deep muscles of the spine, also known as the paravertebral muscles, that run along the length of the spine, the quadratus lumborum and the iliopsoas muscles. These are the muscles that will often seize up and cause your clients to "freeze" or remain unable to stand up straight. They are the muscles that fire when we are in a state of "fight or flight," which is also known as the sympathetic nervous system.

Let's take a look at Mark, whom we have been following throughout the book. If you were treating Mark for the last month and a half or so, you would have learned through open and honest dialogue that he feels unhappy and fearful about his future. He is clearly dissatisfied with his job and continues going to work out of a sense of "responsibility" and also for a feeling of safety and security. His main motivation is to hold on for another five years until he can retire and receive his benefits. This is a decision based on fear. If he had a choice to do anything he wanted to do without any concern for money or retirement security, he would have left long ago. And so he continues to go to a job that he hates, day in and day out, because his fear of not being able to live or survive on income from another source outweighs his desire to be happy and fulfilled in his work. He also feels responsible for his wife who cannot work due to her own illnesses and chronic pain; he feels he has to remain the "strong" one and the provider in the marriage. He holds these feelings deep inside because there is no one he can talk to, and also for fear that he may appear weak and vulnerable.

What does this do to Mark's body? The fear of survival kicks in every day and tightens the muscles around his lower and upper back. He takes in shallow breaths, limiting oxygen flow to his muscles and causing tight knots in the belly of those muscles. He feels somewhat defeated by life, by his responsibilities and obligations, causing his shoulders to round forward and tightening up his anterior chest musculature. This "slouching" posture causes him to push his hips forward as he rests all the weight of his body on his lower back. His hamstrings become tight as he tilts his pelvis in a posterior position. His core and pelvic floor cannot be accessed in this position, so they begin to weaken and he rests all his weight on his lower back.

Each day Mark goes about his business in this state. One day he bends over to pick up something off the floor and his back goes out. He can't stand up straight. All of a sudden he wonders, "What happened? What did I do?"

PRACTICE TIP 15

Have your clients or students ask themselves the following question and listen quietly for their answers. Tell them to be honest with themselves.

"If I had all the money and time in the world, and there were no obstacles, what would I be doing with my life?"

Then get them to ask themselves, "Why am I not doing this?"

Each story is different, but the underlying feelings are the same. There is a sense of deep fear, uncontrollability, and lack of safety and trust in life. To further illustrate this, let us take a look at some of the examples of patients from Chapter 1.

- Lydia's tireless perfectionism came from a deeper lack of self-esteem and a feeling of "not being good enough." The need to control her life was merely a reaction to her lack of inner safety and trust. She grew up with an alcoholic father who was unpredictable and abusive. These emotions manifested in debilitating migraines, shoulder and neck pain, and chronic and often debilitating anxiety.

- Jack had a hard time leaving his lucrative job as a project manager for a construction firm, but always knew deep down he was meant to do something different. He, too, felt afraid of the unknown and often chose the safer path, ignoring his inner calling for something deeper. He struggled with depression and would often find himself isolated and stagnant.

- Simon was young and capable, but was dealing with a great deal of inner anger, fear, and insecurity due to a history of physical abuse as a child. He would often find himself hanging out with the wrong crowd and getting into fights, which led to many injuries and subsequent pain and physical limitations. He knew he was destined to do something better with his life, but he couldn't break the cycle of his destructive patterns.

In *Waking the Tiger* (1997), Peter Levine, founder of the Somatic Experiencing method of healing trauma, explores in detail the effects of trauma on the nervous system and, subsequently, the physical body. He explains how trauma, unless released on a physical level, will get stored in the muscles and tissues. Through observation of animals in the wild, he shows that there is a natural way to release trauma embedded in our physiology. When an animal survives a traumatic event, it has been observed to shake uncontrollably or experience tremors in its muscles. Once the period of "shaking" is over, the animal goes back to its business without holding onto the memory of the trauma. Levine concludes that this reaction is a way to "discharge" stress in the nervous system so that it does not get stored in the body and the nervous system. While animals know how to discharge their trauma naturally, we humans tend to suppress these reactions (as they are deemed socially unacceptable) and often end up with multiple problems later in life, including post-traumatic stress disorder (PTSD).

Berceli, in *The Revolutionary Trauma Release Process* (2008), goes a step further and describes a system and set of exercises that help to induce shaking of the muscles (p.37). Berceli's trauma-releasing exercises bring about this action of shaking, which mimics the natural response that animals experience after a stressful situation. The problem with humans is that we do not allow ourselves to release the trauma on a physical level, so it gets stored in the tissues, only to perpetuate the internal tension. If we keep storing these episodes of trauma without adequate time and space to release, the trauma stays in our system and can wreak havoc on our health and well-being.

As Levine (1997, p.62) writes, "Most modern cultures, including ours, fall victim to the prevailing attitude that strength means endurance; that it is somehow heroic to be able to carry on regardless of the severity of our symptoms." He then goes on to warn us that, "If we attempt to move ahead with our lives, without first yielding to the gentler urges that will guide us back through these harrowing experiences, then our show of strength becomes little more than illusion. In the meantime, the traumatic effects will grow steadily more severe, firmly entrenched and chronic" (p.62).

As I sit here writing this on a rainy day in a Tel Aviv cafe, with a sharp pain in my right shoulder blade and neck extending into my right arm and hand, I am reminded of the work I still need to do in the wake of my father's recent death. I have personally experienced, and continue to experience, the close relationship between unresolved feelings and physical pain.

My personal story

When I first heard of my father's most recent hospitalization, I strongly felt that he was coming to the end of his life. Almost immediately, I experienced tightness and pain in my mid-back area, close to the lower thoracic spine and surrounding muscles. Despite my efforts, my pain did not go away; it persisted throughout the week. When I spoke with my father's doctor in Canada, she explained that, although he had end-stage heart disease, the biggest problem was a backup of fluid due to his weak heart and the increasing load on his failing kidneys.

I was not aware until later that day that my pain was directly over my kidney area. In addition to being the organs that were failing in my father's case, the kidneys are also the organs that hold fear and stress, because the adrenal glands sit just above the kidneys. Most yoga postures that decrease stress and tension and increase energy involve moving the kidneys *into* the body. Back bends (active and restorative) and twists accomplish this. Back bends help us move from the past into the present. By moving the kidneys into the body, we move away from our attachment to how things used to be and move towards being more present in our lives at this moment.

The kidney pain subsided after my father died, but a few days later, as I was sitting with my family at home, I experienced a sudden, shocking pain in my neck and upper back, mostly in my right shoulder blade area. My whole upper body went into spasm and I was unable to move my neck or get up from a supine position without excruciating pain. The only thing that provided relief was doing the Purna Yoga Morning Series and Hip Opening Series. I hadn't done anything to bring on this pain; it was clear to me that this was an emotional reaction manifesting in my body.

Being the oldest in my family of five, I had taken on responsibility for my parents and siblings over the years. The burden of caring for my father had fallen on me because I was home most often and had more resources than my siblings. Pain in the upper back, neck, and shoulders represents a sense of "carrying the weight of the world on your shoulders." An increased sense of responsibility and burden often manifests as tension or pain in this area.

My father's pain

My father's story is a complicated one. At one point in his life he was a prominent rabbi, revered as a brilliant scholar and speaker in our community. And then the tables turned. Events seemed to have shifted in one instant, but in retrospect I can see that there was a slow and steady process that led to his fall from grace. When I was 22, newly married, and in my first year of physical therapy school, my father was arrested on charges of selling drugs to a police officer.

I came to realize that my father, the rabbi, had become involved with a group of crooked individuals who were selling passports, arms, and drugs to make extra money. My family and I had no knowledge of his involvement, but as the days unfolded, we learned that he was trying to support our family in maintaining our then upper-middle-class suburban status, despite having lost his most recent job.

How does someone in such a powerful and prestigious position sink so low? I have asked myself that question over and over again as I struggle to put the pieces together for myself. What I recall most often are my father's strong beliefs. His *samskaras*, or patterns of experience and psychological conditioning, were such that he did not trust others, and often felt unappreciated and unseen. He sometimes sabotaged relationships with friends and co-workers by being sharp or unkind, perhaps to disguise his feelings of hurt and sadness. He was not supported by my mother, who demanded that he fulfill the traditional role of the Jewish father and support us financially while she tended to the home and children. He felt alone, isolated. He closed off his heart to those closest to him.

After the discovery of his crime and his jail time was served, he retreated to a simple studio apartment, exiled and depressed. He lost contact with the community and with all his children. I believe he felt that we were better off without him in our lives. But we felt hurt and abandoned and ran further away from him.

Physically, my father was not a sick man, but his public exposure and alienation from his family marked the beginning of his mental and physical decline. He did have a heart condition, but I believe he aged prematurely from carrying his shame and negativity inside. When discussing his health, his doctor told me that "your father's heart is working at 15 percent of capacity." I remember thinking how appropriate that statement was, for the heart was his weak area. He didn't know how to use his heart any more than that.

I now realize that he did the best he could. His father had died when he was 15 years old and he was raised in a family that did not express love or emotions freely. He tried to be a good father, a good husband, and to provide, but he felt he failed. And ultimately, he surrendered to sadness and shame. He was unable to see—beyond his own pain—the love that existed around him. Our family was ready to embrace him, had he just asked.

Carrying the weight of the world

Being the oldest, and the only one of the older children living in town at the time of his arrest, I spent some days in court watching the trial unfold, other days with my mother trying to save the house from foreclosure, and still other days going to jail to visit my father and bring him cigarettes, bagels, and knishes. I also took care of my brother, inviting him to dinner or letting him spend weekends because he was having such a hard time emotionally. I tried to be there for everyone. My schooling and my marriage suffered because I was overwhelmed, lonely, and lost emotionally myself.

My parents divorced and I became the only one who could visit my father in jail. On one particular visit I asked him to tell me the truth, to be open with me about what happened. I felt that if I was shouldering so much responsibility, the least he could do was open up to me. He stared at me with a blank look on his face and told me at that moment that he never wanted to see me again.

I learned then that if I express my truth or ask for something I need, I will be rejected. That lesson has haunted me to this day. True or not, that conclusion came from my experience. I did not speak to my father for ten years after that.

After being immersed in yoga for a number of years, I finally called my father again, breaking our silence. I knew that the anger and hurt I carried only hurt me. To be kind to myself I had to make peace with him. He remained cold but was open to talking. He was living isolated in his studio apartment, working for a bagel shop and old age home on the side. A year later, I received a call that he had had a stroke.

I flew back to Montreal to discover that, once again, my father was in need of help. With no one else to step up, I was thrust into the role of case manager, and when we realized that my father's short-term memory and cognition were severely affected by the stroke, I had to terminate his lease, sell his car, clean out his apartment, and sort out his financial documents as we transitioned him into a nursing care facility.

Years went by. I would visit at least once a year and found myself having to buy him new clothes, socks, and underwear at each visit; no one else took care of that. I felt sad to experience this role reversal, to realize that I was now picking out my once brilliant and bold father's underwear in a discount store.

Soon after his death, I experienced that same sense of responsibility without feeling the closeness and the love. When I arrived from Israel, I had to go to the hospital to sign a release, see the body, and proceed to make funeral arrangements, including applying for government assistance with the funeral expenses. My father had not prepared for this day, and so, once again, the onus was on us, his children, to organize and finance his final ceremony.

The pain in my right shoulder blade and neck is still there. I believe its roots lie in this story. Day by day I work on my meditation and yoga practice with the intention of seeing where this pain comes from and helping to release it little by little. It is getting better, but the layers run deep and I know it will take some time. But ignoring it will only allow the pain to continue. The first step is to see and recognize it. Only then can I hope to let it go.

Achieving this release is the work of yoga, especially its second branch, the Niyamas or personal practices; these include *Tapas* (discipline and zeal), *Svadhyaya* (self-study), and *Ishvaripranidhana* (surrender). I feel so lucky to have yoga's roadmap guiding me towards wholeness and continued growth. I can stop my father's legacy here and now, and find a way for my heart to work at 100 percent of capacity, one beat and one breath at a time.

My yoga teacher, Aadil Palkhivala, tells a story about a day when he was traveling with his family and had to stop at a railroad track to wait for a train to pass by. At the railroad crossing, he got out of the car to watch the train go by. An older gentleman one car behind got out of his vehicle as well and walked over to Aadil. As the train approached, the man began to speak to my teacher. The noise of the train became louder and Aadil could not hear what the man was saying, but did not want to appear rude. He nodded politely and smiled back at the man. Satisfied, the man got back into his car just as the train made its way towards its next stop.

About half a mile down the road, Aadil came to a fork in the road and made a left turn as he was accustomed to. A few minutes later, he heard a loud "pop," and he slowed down, realizing that his tire was flat. When he got out of the car, he noticed that broken glass all over the road had caused the puncture in the tire.

It was then that it occurred to him. The older gentleman at the train tracks had gotten out of his car to tell him that there had been an accident earlier and was warning him to avoid that particular road due to the broken glass from the wreck. However, since the noise of the train was so loud, he could not hear what the man was saying. Had he been able to hear the warning, Aadil might have been able to go a different route and avoid the flat tire altogether.

At the end of the story, my teacher paused. Then he said, "The older gentleman in the story represents your heart. The train represents the noise in your mind. The work of yoga is to quiet the noise in the mind so that you can listen to the soft whisper of your heart's longing."

This is the work of yoga. While the various physical postures can benefit the spine and lengthen the hamstrings, the ultimate intention of the practice is to train the mind and harness the ego, so that we can hear what our hearts are telling us. Then it is up to us to listen.

I have seen many clients over the years who have been diligent with their exercises, but continue to experience chronic tension and pain in their bodies. What is often revealed when we go deeper is that there is a conflict between their will or intellect and their heart. Many find themselves in destructive or unhealthy relationships or jobs that are not feeding their souls. There may be unresolved trauma or grief that needs to be addressed. When we introduce the deeper aspects of the practice, magic happens. Not only does their pain resolve, they often find themselves naturally making changes in their lives, impacting their overall level of contentment and satisfaction. Strangely enough, this happens with little effort. It's amazing what happens when we get out of our own way.

What are these mysterious "deeper levels of practice"? Are they accessible to anyone or only to the ascetic who sits way up high in the Himalayas?

The answer is simple. If you can breathe, you can do yoga. We will go over some simple pranayama and meditation techniques that you can add to your students' home program.

Pranayama: Getting started

"Prana" is translated as *breath* or *life force*, while "yama" refers to *regulation and control*. Pranayama therefore refers to the regulation of life force through the breath or, as it is often translated, "mastery of the life force." Breathing is unique in that it is a function that is involuntary, yet can be controlled and changed by voluntary action as well. The breath also connects our mind directly to our body and, more importantly, to our nervous system.

Most of us, after waking up to a loud alarm clock, pounding a cup or two of coffee down our throats, getting the kids off to school, watching the morning news, checking our email and voice messages, and driving to work in rush hour traffic, may notice that our nervous system is in a state of stress. What has happened is that our sympathetic nervous system, the one that tells us we are in a state of "fight or flight," is activated; this sets off a chain of events that includes an increase in breathing and heart rate, increased muscular tension, and dilated pupils. Your body does not know the difference if you are late for an important meeting or if you are running away from a hungry tiger; the physiological effects are the same. Stress in any form turns up the heat.

Conversely, after a quiet walk in the forest on a vacation day, your nervous system may be in a state of rest and calm. This is due to the activation of the parasympathetic nervous system, which is the state we want to be in most of the day. If we are not in a state of panic or stress, our breathing and heart rate is slow and regular, our digestion begins to work, healing of injuries can take place, our muscles can relax, and the body can focus on reproduction. We are calm, relaxed, and focused.

One of the aims of the pranayama exercises below is to teach your students or clients how to breathe correctly so that the body shifts from the sympathetic (fight or flight) state to the parasympathetic state. Just as stress can cause us to breathe faster, we can manipulate our breathing to relieve stress. The more your clients practice these simple techniques regularly, the more you will see them create an optimal state for healing to occur, as they also quiet their minds just enough to connect with their hearts.

In the practice tip below are several important suggestions to convey to your students or clients when helping them begin their pranayama practice:

PRACTICE TIP 16

- *Don't judge what comes up when you are breathing*. The mind is tricky and will get bored, angry, impatient, and anxious and will not stop thinking. Know this before you start: *It is completely normal!* Your job is just to continue to redirect your mind to your breathing, even if you must do so every single second.

- *Practice acceptance*. As thoughts arise, you may find that many of the feelings that arise are uncomfortable. You are not your thoughts. Just observe them as you would for an outsider, and accept them. Sometimes I speak to my thoughts, saying, "Ah, there you are. I see you." Recognize these feelings, acknowledge them, and then let them go.

- *Practice for at least six months consistently*. The results of a pranayama practice are not immediate. In fact, it is a lifetime practice. In my experience, you can start to feel the effects of a consistent practice after six months, so keep going until then, even if your ego tries to convince you to stop. The dishes and emails will always be there. Give yourself this gift.

Pranayama is a very powerful tool. This is why it is important that your students or clients practice under the guidance of a teacher, and that they be wary of teachers who throw out random pranayama exercises in the middle of class. Often they do not know why they are doing it and how it will impact their students. Remember that pranayama is the fourth limb of yoga and follows asana (physical postures). The order of the limbs is important, as you can have an asana practice without any pranayama, but in order to practice pranayama, you must have a regular asana practice. The asana practice helps build strength both physically and in the nervous system, so that the student has enough strength and resilience to hold the prana. Like an electrical outlet, the student's nervous system can only take so much of a pranic charge. If the voltage is too high, it can blow out the student's nervous system.

I am introducing pranayama techniques to you that my teacher, Aadil Palkhivala, taught to me. Aadil emphasizes that most of us are "vata imbalanced" in our society. This means that we are overstimulated and our nervous systems are overactive and unable to rest. Therefore it is more beneficial for beginners to work on pranayama that calms the nervous system and has a grounding effect. (Incidentally, I consider an individual who has been practicing pranayama for under ten years a beginner.) Stimulating breath work such as *kapalabhati* (breath of fire) or long holds should be practiced under the guidance of a personal teacher only.

Teaching beginning pranayama

When teaching individuals who have never had a breathing practice before, it is important to work on a few points first:

- *Begin pranayama in a supine position.* In order to access the diaphragm as the main muscle of respiration, it is best to begin breathing while lying down. When seated it is harder to turn off the neck muscles, namely the upper trapezius, scalenes, and sternocleidomastoid. For those who have not learned how to breathe properly, it is best to facilitate relaxation of the neck muscles by lying down. Once they get comfortable with diaphragmatic breathing, they can move to a seated position to practice pranayama.

- *Teach belly breathing first.* Belly breathing is not true pranayama, but it is a *prerequisite* for pranayama. You will need to teach a beginner how to use their diaphragm, the major muscle of respiration, instead of the neck muscles, the accessory muscles of respiration.

- *Teach them how to activate the POA (pit of the abdomen).* Many new practitioners have no idea how to access their lower belly, which is essential for pranayama. Use techniques such as manual cuing in order to teach them how to engage the belly without gripping or holding the breath.

- *Emphasize the proper way to inhale/exhale.* Most people will suck their bellies in when they inhale. You will need to work with them so they can learn how to allow the belly to rise on the inhalation, and how to draw the navel towards the spine on the exhalation. This is the way to breathe during asana practice as well.

Positioning

Positioning is extremely important to obtain the desired effect—a relaxed nervous system. Pay close attention to detail. If one aspect is out of alignment, your student may not be able to reach a state where the parasympathetic nervous system can be activated. You want your student or client to be lying supine over a bolster or blanket folded as a rectangle under the back.

Instruct your student to lie lengthwise over the bolster, with the buttocks a few inches away from the bolster. The bolster should be under the lower ribs, but not the lower back. *The main intention is for the belly to move towards the legs and for the lungs to move towards the head, thereby freeing up the diaphragm to breathe more freely.*

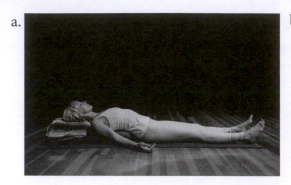
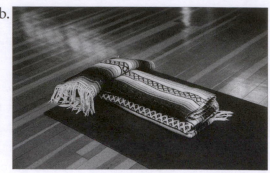

Figure 8.1 Proper position for supine pranayama: a. on bolster; b. blanket set-up

Place a blanket folded up neatly under the head, so that the back of the head (occiput) is supported and the chin is slightly tucked towards the center of the chest, and so that the gaze is towards the heart center. Ask the student to gaze internally towards the chest with soft eyes and to rest the tongue on the bottom palate. In yoga, we keep the mouth closed and breathe in and out through the nostrils only. Keep the eyes and eyelids soft and relaxed.

1. Belly breathing–preparation for pranayama

Most of the clients you see will be breathing incorrectly. They will often be contracting their neck muscles and sucking the belly in on inhalation. Belly breathing should be practiced until they can comfortably breathe while sitting, using the diaphragm only.

In a supine pranayama position, have the client lie down and start by placing her hands on her belly. On the inhalation, the belly should rise. This shows her that the diaphragm is descending and pushing the abdominal contents forward.

Watch your client's face and make sure that she is relaxed and that the neck muscles are not activated. On the exhalation, the belly should fall as the diaphragm recoils back up into the rib cage.

Ask your client to practice belly breathing for five minutes twice a day in supine for a few weeks. Once your client can do this comfortably, have them attempt the same exercise in a sitting position. Make sure they pay attention to the belly rising and falling only, and release any tension or activation in the neck muscles.

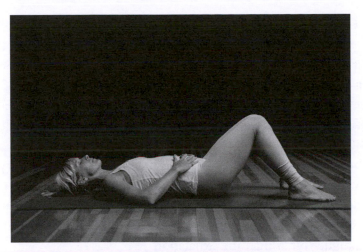

Figure 8.2 Belly breathing—supine

2. Movement of the lungs and rib cage

At the beginning, inhale fully into the lungs so that the lungs inflate towards the ribs. Once they are almost in contact, expand the ribs at the same rate as the lungs, with the space between them remaining constant, until the inhalation is complete.

Note: If the ribs do not expand but the lungs do, the student needs more back bends. If the rib cage expands but the lungs do not fill, the student needs more pranayama.

On the exhalation, let the rib cage and lungs deflate at the same rate until the rib cage comes back to its resting position. Then continue to exhale with the lungs until the exhalation is complete.

Practice this for five to ten minutes daily.

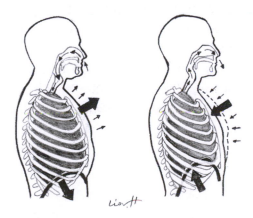

Figure 8.3 Movement of the lungs and rib cage during pranayama

3. Ujjayi breathing

Ujjayi is a very good breathing practice to begin with. Remember that it is not better if it is louder. The aim of this breath is to be soft and smooth.

You can begin teaching this technique by using the exhalation first. Tell your student to inhale through the nose, and exhale, making a "Ha" sound in the back of the throat. Use the image of fogging up the car window with your breath as an illustration of the quality of the "Ha" sound.

Once the student is comfortable with this sound, he or she can try it with the mouth closed. That will create the "H" sound in the back of the throat.

Then add the inhalation. The inhalation is described as an "S" sound as in "So." It feels as if you are inhaling through an imaginary hole in your throat, and it has a higher pitch than the exhalation.

Make sure the POA is slightly engaged and practice the Ujjayi breath, filling up the chest cavity with breath on the inhalation, and releasing on the exhalation. The POA is engaged during both inhalation and exhalation, but much more so during the exhalation.

Practice for five to ten minutes.

Make sure your client takes a 5- to 15-minute Savasana after any pranayama practice. This cannot be omitted.

4. Three-part breathing in sitting

Have your client sit up on a cushion or bolster so that the spine is in a neutral position. Tell him to place his hands on his lower ribs (one hand on each side) and inhale, filling up the lower lungs with breath. Repeat for 15 breaths.

Then move the hands to the middle rib cage area, underneath the armpits, and take 15 breaths, filling up the middle lungs so that the ribs move out into your hands on each inhalation.

Finally, have the client place his hands on the upper chest area, so the shoulders do not rise, and complete 15 deep breaths, focusing on filling the upper lungs with breath.

If your client finds his mind wandering, tell him to bring it back to the area on which he is focusing. Have him notice how he can move the breath into different areas of his body with his awareness.

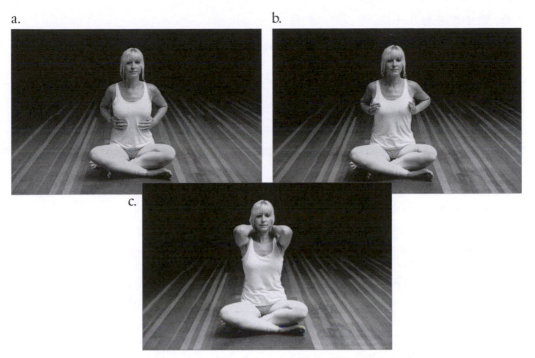

Figure 8.4 Three-part breathing: a. lower lungs; b. middle lungs; c. upper lungs

5. Nadi Shodhana (alternate nostril breathing)

Practice Nadi Shodhana in a seated position with the spine erect. Place the thumb just above the right nostril and the ring finger just above the left nostril. Take one full breath in and one out, before beginning the practice.

Gently close off the right nostril and inhale through the left nostril. Then close the left nostril off with the ring finger, and exhale through the right nostril. Take an inhalation through the right nostril, close it off and exhale though the left. Inhale left, close it off, and exhale right.

Repeat this pattern, beginning and ending on the left side (in order to activate the parasympathetic nervous system).

Keep the breath quiet and even. You can imagine creating the shape of the infinity symbol with your breath as it moves smoothly from right to left. Do not hold the breath here.

This technique is especially good for calming the fluctuations of the mind and creating mental stability.

For depression: Breathe in and out with the right nostril only.

For anxiety: Breathe through the left nostril only.

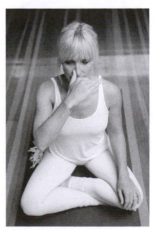

Figure 8.5 Nadi Shodhana (alternate nostril breathing)

6. Viloma I, II, III

This technique can be practiced both sitting and supine, initially under close supervision by the teacher. Have your client start in supine, as it is easier to accomplish this breathing technique without activating the neck muscles. Once practiced for a few months, clients can try it in a seated position.

There are three types of Viloma:

a.   *Viloma I*—interrupted inhalation

b.   *Viloma II*—interrupted exhalation

c.   *Viloma III*—interrupted inhalation and exhalation.

a. Viloma I

Inhale in three equal parts, pausing between each inhalation. Then exhale fully without any pauses. Begin by inhaling for two seconds and pausing for two seconds; then breathe in again for two seconds and pause for two seconds. Complete one more round of inhalation for two seconds and pause for two seconds, and then exhale fully for 12 seconds (a. in Figure 8.6).

This technique is good for depression and lethargy.

b. Viloma II

Take one complete inhalation, and exhale in three parts, pausing in between each partial exhalation. Begin by taking a deep inhalation for 12 seconds. Then exhale for two seconds and pause for two seconds, and repeat this pattern two more times for a total of three rounds (b. in Figure 8.6).

This technique is good for anxiety and scattered thinking.

c. Viloma III

Inhale in three parts, exhale in three parts (c. in Figure 8.6). Make sure the amount of time spent inhaling and pausing are of equal duration.

This technique is good for balance.

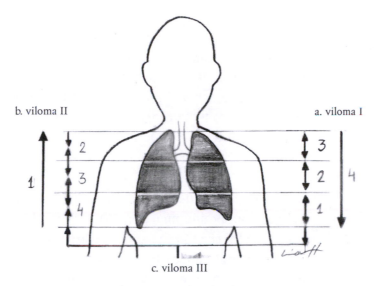

Figure 8.6 Viloma breathing

7. Bhamari breath

This technique is very easy and can be done anywhere at any time. It translates to "humming bee breath," because it sounds like a swarm of bees buzzing in the distance.

Have the student inhale deeply, and on the exhalation keep the lips close together and allow the escaping air to make a deep buzzing/humming sound in the sinus cavity, radiating into the body so it sounds like a swarm of bees far away.

This is extremely calming and good for anxiety, stress, insomnia, and overall relaxation.

Meditation: Getting started

Meditation may be both the easiest and most difficult thing you will ever do—or teach your clients how to do—in your life. It really is as simple as sitting, breathing, and continuously bringing your attention back to your breath. But somehow the ability to stop what we are doing and sit for even 10 to 15 minutes may seem impossible. If we all know that meditating can offer us more peace and calm in this unsettling world, why don't we do it more often? After all, it is completely free and available to us anytime and anywhere.

If only it were that easy. Our minds are constantly at work trying to keep us busy being worried. Why? It really comes back to our built-in survival instincts and our basic physiology. Because our nervous systems are built for survival, like animals in the wild we are constantly on guard for danger and wired to worry about our safety and security. What makes us different from animals, however, is that we have the ability to retrain our brain so that our responses to external and internal stimuli are different from theirs. This does not happen by itself. In order to change thought patterns, reactions, and even our response to stress, we need to access the potential of *neuroplasticity*. Pascual-Leone *et al.* (2011) define neuroplasticity, also known as brain plasticity, as "changes in neural pathways and synapses due to changes in behavior, environment, neural processes, thinking, emotions, as well as changes resulting from bodily injury" (p.302). What this means is that direct *experience* can actually change the way our brain functions. The key to accomplishing this seemingly impossible task is through *repetition*. In order for our brain to learn how to process things and react differently, a new pathway needs to be created which requires a type of re-patterning that can only come from consistent practice. After time, the response will become automatic.

For example, when my friends come late to a party I have been planning for a while, I notice that I begin to get angry with them, so that by the time they arrive, I cannot enjoy their company. If I inquire deeply, I can see that their showing up late triggers a belief that I have from childhood, something that is painful and brings up an array of emotions including sadness, loneliness, and grief. What it reinforces are feelings that "I am not important enough," "no one cares about me," and "the people I trust most will eventually leave and abandon me." Somehow in my brain there is an automatic connection between their tardiness and my importance to them, which sends me into a loop of deep anger and resentment. But what I really feel underneath it all is sadness and grief for the little girl who was ignored and never told she was important and worthy of unconditional love.

Yoga gives us the ability to slow down and pay attention to these deeper belief systems. Instead of becoming reactive, I may choose to sit with the pain for a moment, acknowledge it, and really *feel* it. Then I may decide to tell myself another story, such as: "My friends care about me, they are just running late, and it has nothing to do with my level of importance to them or their commitment to our friendship." The feeling of anger will not go away after this one time, but if I keep repeating this message to myself every time there is a similar occurrence, eventually those strong emotions will no longer be triggered.

Below you will find some basics of Heartfull™ Meditation, created by Savitri, aimed at changing patterns of thought and consequently, behavior. When practiced regularly, your clients will feel more peaceful, accepting of life on its terms and supported by something greater than themselves. They begin to rest in this understanding and their pain, both physical and emotional, will diminish. Included are two techniques to introduce you to the beauty of Heartfull Meditation. There are many other additional Heartfull Meditation techniques that are also available from Savitri, to open the heart chakra, create a protective energy field, lift pelvic energy, etc.

Heartfull™ Meditation Snacks/Techniques[1]

These meditation "snacks" come directly from Heartfull™ Meditation created by Savitri (2015) and are quoted from Savitri with permission for you to share with your students or clients.

Please note: It is recommended that you practice these techniques regularly for at least six months before teaching them to anyone.

All techniques can be done sitting or standing, preferably with your eyes closed to deepen the experience of feeling beautiful feelings that are the true you.

1. Eternal Breath (24/7)

The intention is to bring more Light (your true Self, your Spirit) into your body.

a. Wherever you are, feel the air around you glowing in White Light with the feeling of pure love.

b. Whenever you inhale, imagine White Light entering your nostrils and flowing into your brain and eyes. When you exhale, let go of your thoughts, tensions, worries, exhaustion, confusion, etc. out through your nostrils (or through your slightly open mouth). Know that these thoughts, tensions, worries, etc. are your ego, and feel them going back to White Light (the Divine in everything) to be healed.

c. As you exhale, think "I offer _____ to the White Light in the universe to be healed." This helps clarify your intention. As you inhale, think "I welcome truth, joy, and love into my life."

---

1   © Copyright 2016, Heartfull™ Meditation, by Savitri, all rights reserved. Do not copy, reproduce, or alter.

Do this as often as possible during the day to feel connected with your Spirit and to help release old habits. This will calm the mind and the nervous system. Remember that the Light is your true eternal Self.

2. Centering Mental Energy (1½ minutes)

The intention is to bring the past (left brain) and future (right brain), as well as your senses, into the now (the Heart Chakra). Imagine a straight line through the center of the mind and body to the center of the Heart Chakra.

a. With your eyes closed, place your hands with your fingers together and slightly cupped, on the right and left sides of your head, facing your ears. Your hands should be approximately three inches away from your head.

b. Exhaling, bring your hands together in Namaste, not more than one inch away from your face, with the tips of your thumbs at the same level as the eyebrows.

c. Inhale, and then on the next exhalation bring your hands down *slowly* to your Heart Chakra. As you do this, make your mind follow a straight line in the center of your body (the Pillar of Light), offering your mind to your heart.

d. Think "I offer my mind and senses to my soul within" or "I offer my mind and senses to my heart, to my soul, where joy, love, and wisdom await me." Stay a few moments at the Heart Chakra and feel the mind turning inward.

e. Do a–d three times.

Use this technique when you have too many thoughts, are tired of living in the mind, feel unfocused, overwhelmed, confused, scattered, ungrounded, angry, annoyed, or tired, are daydreaming or when your eyes and forehead are tense and painful. This technique is beneficial when you have trouble relaxing your mind, body, or eyes. Centering helps you to fall asleep. It brings your awareness back into your body, into the safe place where your soul resides. It is extremely useful for staying centered and being aware of your body while doing asana or any form of exercise. It helps prevent injuries, since injuries only happen when we are unaware or unfocused.

PRACTICE TIP 17

After meditation or pranayama, have your clients ask themselves the questions below and write down the answers in a journal. It is helpful for them to take a long, hard look at the deeper aspects of their beliefs that may be affecting their pain and impacting the quality of their lives. The more they are willing to take a look at these beliefs, the less they will have control over them. This is not an easy process, but well worth the effort.

Reassure them that they do not have to do anything with these answers. They are just for reading over and acknowledging. Have your clients notice how the answers make them feel. Ask them where they feel sensations in their body when they take a look at what is really going on inside. Then they can take a few deep breaths and just say, "I see you." Instruct them to let the beliefs know that you are willing to observe them and acknowledge them, but that they are just that—beliefs; they are not necessarily the Truth—your Truth.

Questions for journaling:

- What beliefs are limiting you in your life?
- Where in your life do you feel out of control?
- Do you feel a lack of support in your life?
- Do you carry anger/resentment? At what or whom?
- Is money or security a source of anxiety for you?

CASE STUDY: MARK

Treatment Session 6

Mark has been progressing well with his program and he now has a solid understanding of his home exercise program. He is feeling a great deal better—almost 80 percent—and is happy with the improvement. But often he notices that the pain is worse in the morning right before he goes to work, and diminishes on the weekends. I ask him to be honest and to tell me why he thinks his pain is worse in the morning and at work. (Notice that I like to ask questions and listen, rather than insert my point of view here. It is not my job to tell him about his emotional landscape, as I do not know what is going on in every aspect of his life. What I can do is use my intuition, developed through personal practice and my own journey, to ask him the right questions.)

After a few minutes, Mark broke down. He confessed to me that he gets nervous before going in to work because he truly dislikes his job and many of the people surrounding him in the office. He feels so much pressure to provide for his wife and son that he grits his teeth and bears all the nonsense he has to face every day with one thing in mind—his pension when he retires in five years. So basically, every day, he wakes up and goes to a job he hates because of fear. He feels out of control and that he does everything for everyone else and ignores his own needs and desires. He does not feel supported by his family and has no one to talk to about his desperation. He spends a few minutes letting the tears flow in my office. I tell him that it is all right to cry and that he should not hold anything back. I create a safe space where he can be heard without any judgment.

There is the old thought that maybe I am wasting his session time as we are not doing any physical exercises, and after all, this is physical therapy. But then I tell myself that *this is the real work of yoga*. That we are getting to the heart of the matter and the reason for all his internal gripping and tension.

Towards the end of our session, I offer him some meditation and pranayama tools to practice every morning. For now, it is too frightening for him to leave his job as a solution, but we can change his relationship to having to go to his job each day.

I give Mark the following tools to practice every day:

- Five minutes of three-part breathing. This helps him learn how to direct his breath into different areas of his body and to relax the tension in the trunk musculature. It is also very calming and soothing for the nervous system.

- The Heartfull™ Medtation snacks. He does the breathing and mental centering technique. I ask him to really focus on what his heart is longing for, so that he can discover what it is he really wants to do with his life, and I encourage him to nourish himself by doing things he loves, such as walking along the beach with his wife.

- Next I have him focus on something or someone he is grateful for in his life. Focusing on gratitude is the single best way to fight depression, as it creates a state of mind that is positive and peaceful. We all should try it, for it is impossible to focus on what you are grateful for and be upset at the same time.

- Finally, I work with Mark to find a mantra (or saying) to repeat to himself at the end of his ten-minute meditation. He decides on "I am supported and receive everything I need each day. I am loved."

At this point, we have covered a multifaceted approach towards healing from back pain using Purna Yoga and the kosha model. We have addressed the physical body (*annamaya kosha*) through its stages of healing with solid, alignment-based, therapeutic techniques. You have seen how to connect your clients or students with their energetic bodies (*pranamaya kosha*) by developing awareness and modulation of the breath—first during the postures, and later with more specific pranayama techniques. The mental or emotional body (*manomaya kosha*) was explored through inquiry and mindfulness practice during the postures, pranayama, meditation, and journaling, and through focused awareness throughout the day. And finally, we identified the intellect or belief systems (*vijnanamaya kosha*) that we carry as "our story" by quieting the body and mind, using all the techniques listed in order to create some space to see how all of our reactions are shaping our reality each and every day. What we hope for, as a result of this approach, is that we can help our clients or students achieve a sustained experience of Bliss (*anandamaya kosha*); in that place, they will be able to rest in contentment, regardless of external circumstances, and let go both physically and emotionally.

We have also worked through the five stages of healing, which are the following:

1. *Realign:* Identify what is tight and what is weak and work on correcting both.

2. *Create space:* Open up the tight structures and surrounding connective tissue to reduce joint and nerve compression.

3. *Re-educate:* Identify faulty movement patterns that contribute to the imbalances, and so clients and students can learn how to move in a different way.

4. *Stabilize:* Once the structure is aligned, then help stabilize it.

5. *Practice:* Be consistent for long-term results and transformation. Guide your students to make their practice a good habit, like brushing their teeth.

In Part II you will learn ways to design effective classes for back health, including intelligent sequencing, as well as teaching styles and themes to explore with your students. My aim is to bring all the information together into a class context to make you a more knowledgeable, skilled, effective, and intuitive teacher. I have also included recommended sequences for various conditions. It is my hope that this work will help you and your clients and students find a new way to approach the healing process, using yoga as therapy for a much happier back and also a healthier, more integrated self.

PART II

Teaching Yoga for a Happy Back

CHAPTER 9

Sequencing and the Art of Teaching

Incorrect instructions for healthy students may be correct instructions for therapeutics. Know the difference.

Aadil Palkhivala

Teaching is both a science and an art. It is one thing to be a yoga student and take hundreds of classes, but the moment you stand at the front of the room, your world changes entirely. Left is right and right is left. Both beginners and advanced practitioners are looking to you to guide them, as well as people with knee problems, shoulder injuries, and, of course, back pain. In fact, the more you actually learn about the body and yoga, the harder it becomes to teach a group class, for you come to realize that each pose should be adapted differently to each individual. Have you noticed that as a beginning teacher you were a lot more confident than you are now, with a little (or a lot) more knowledge under your belt? If that is the case, you are most likely on the right track. Even more challenging than teaching such varied groups is designing classes for individuals with back pain; everyone is experiencing different symptoms and each person comes to class with his or her own needs.

While the task might seem overwhelming, it is indeed possible. For those with complicated conditions, I always recommend at least one private session to see whether they are good candidates for group classes. Such a person may need to do some private work to get prepared to join a class eventually, especially if there is limitation due to pain or neurological symptoms. *The aim of a "Yoga for a Happy Back" class is to teach groups how to prevent back pain and to encourage healing from generalized back pain caused by postural problems.* Classes are not a substitute for private and personalized treatment by a healthcare professional, but should be used as an adjunct when appropriate. This decision should be made on a case-by-case basis.

When designing effective classes, the first thing to do is to look at common trends in individuals who have back pain and at postures that help everyone, no matter their conditions. The following class themes tend to benefit anyone struggling with lower back pain. While we cannot be absolutely specific to each person's condition when teaching a group, these class ideas should help meet the needs of the general public.

Yoga for a Happy Back class themes

1. Hamstrings openers

Most individuals with lower back pain tend to have tight hamstrings, which pull the pelvis into a posterior tilt, thereby decreasing the lumbar curve. There are a number of yoga postures that stretch the hamstrings and can be very helpful for your students, especially those who sit in chairs for a number of hours each day at work. The best postures to include in this class are: Supta Padangusthasana (reclining hand to big toe pose) with variations; Half-Uttanasana (standing forward bend) at the wall; Parsvottanasana (pyramid pose) at the wall, with hands on blocks; Trikonasana (triangle pose); and a Prasarita Padottanasana (standing wide-legged forward fold).

Note: Even though full forward bends tend to stretch the hamstrings, we want to avoid such full folds, especially those deeper ones in which the legs are close together as in Paschimottanasana (seated forward fold) or Full Uttanasana (standing forward fold), for these are contraindicated for individuals with a herniated or bulging disc. In my Happy Back classes, I assume that everyone has a herniated disc and so I only teach postures that are safe for all individuals. (If someone has stenosis or spondylolisthesis, I caution them not to do full back bends, as spinal extension is contraindicated for these conditions; but I do have them practice the actions of back bends in neutral—these include relaxing the shoulder blades down, internal rotation of the thighs, relaxing the buttocks, opening the chest, etc.)

a.

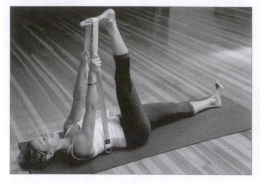

b.

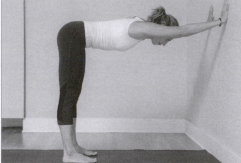

c.

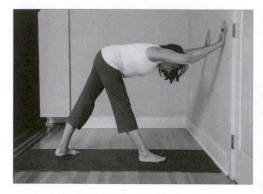

d.

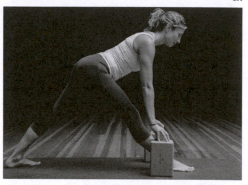

Figure 9.1 Hamstring sequence:
a. lying on the ground lifting right leg up with a strap
b. Half-Uttanasana at the wall
c. hands on the wall with one leg forward
d. with hands on blocks
e. Trikonasana
f. Prasarita Padottanasana

e.

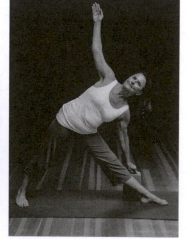

f.

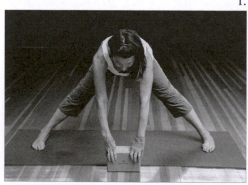

2. Psoas openers

As we discussed in previous chapters, the psoas is an area that tends to be tight and goes into spasm when there is tension in the body and in the mind. It is the muscle that corresponds to the sympathetic (fight or flight) nervous system and pulls the spine into excessive lordosis when tight. It can also cause compression by pulling a vertebral segment into rotation when one side is tighter than the other. Opening and allowing the psoas to release helps *everyone*. The individuals who especially benefit are the overly flexible yoga students and teachers who tend to overextend their spines during their yoga practice. Because this muscle is so deep, stretching it will not feel the same to you and your students as other common stretches. The work of opening the psoas is much more subtle. Those Type A personalities (you know who you are!) tend to want to feel an intense stretch of some sort—but the psoas needs patience, longer holds, and a great deal of focus on the breath in order to release. Poses that are helpful for achieving that release include lunges with longer holds and an emphasis on lifting the POA (pit of the abdomen); internal rotation from the hip series Virabhadrasana I (warrior I); and variations, whether with the hands on the wall, the heel up on the wall, or with the front thigh supported on a chair.

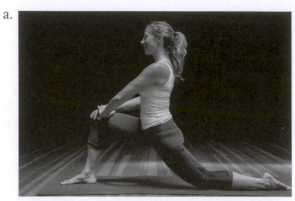

a.

Figure 9.2 Psoas openers:
a. supported lunge
b. internal rotation from the hip series
c. Virabhadrasana I
d. hands at the wall
e. the heel up on the wall
f. with the front thigh supported on a chair

b.

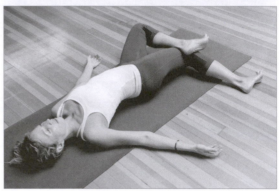

c.

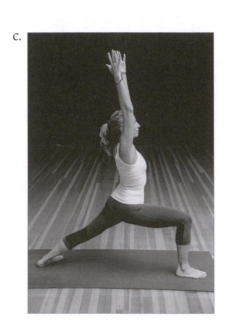

d.

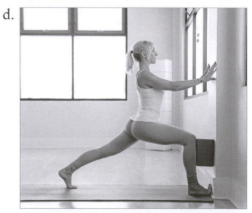

e.

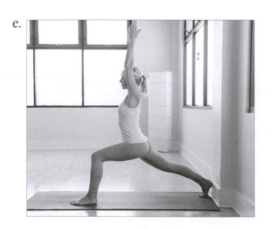

f.

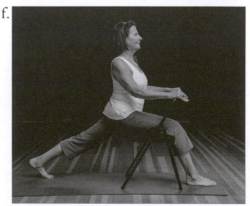

3. All hip openers

The key to relieving back pain lies in opening tight muscles around the pelvis and hip. The Purna Yoga Hip Opening Series is one of the most valuable sequences for those struggling with lower back pain. Since the hip muscles exert a pull on the pelvis, any imbalance will directly affect the mobility of the lumbar spine. Keeping the hips in balance is important to prevent unequal forces on the spine and surrounding structures.

Sometimes external rotation poses, such as Baddha Konasana (butterfly pose) or Supta Baddha Konasana (reclining butterfly pose), cause more discomfort in individuals with lower back pain, due to sacroiliac joint dysfunction. You can design an entire class based on the hip series with adjustments, or you can use the hip series as a warm-up and opening for the class to prepare students for other postures.

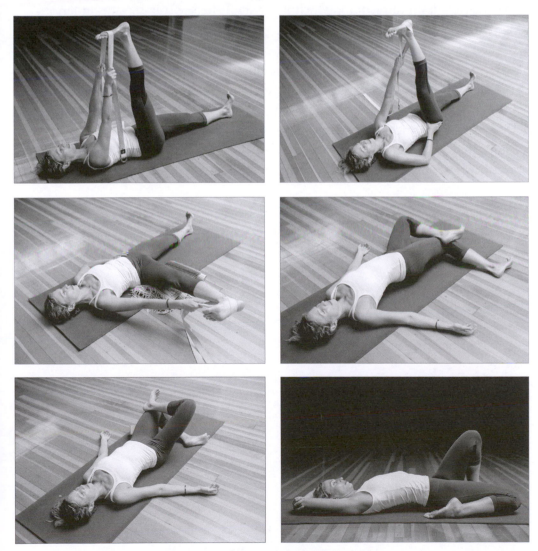

Figure 9.3 The Purna Yoga Hip Opening Series

4. Shoulder blade stabilizers

Many individuals with back pain have very little knowledge of how to access their shoulder blades, and how important the actions of the scapulae are to facilitate an efficient and tension-free posture. My teacher has always encouraged me to teach with the intention of giving students a new awareness or understanding of their bodies. You might begin by explaining to your students where the shoulder blades are. Teach them what you mean when you say, "Move the shoulder blades away from the ears," or "Spread the shoulder blades apart." It is likely that they do not know how to do that in their bodies. Tracing the actions of the shoulder blades with your index finger is a very effective way of letting the student know what to activate. Encourage the descent of the shoulder blades, which requires the activation of the lower trapezius muscle and the action of spreading or wrapping of the shoulder blades (protraction), which is accomplished by the serratus anterior muscle. These are the two movements required in many yoga postures and are needed to encourage the natural spinal curves. In addition, activation of the serratus anterior muscle causes a relaxation response in the upper trapezius and levator scapulae muscles, helping to relieve neck tension and pain in the cervical region. Poses that encourage the descent and spreading of the shoulder blades include: Tadasana, Half-Uttanasana, preparation for plank, Supported Chaturanga (with chest on a bolster), downward-facing dog, Prasarita Padottanasana, and forearm plank pose.

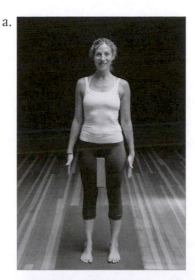

Figure 9.4 Shoulder blade sequence:
a. Tadasana
b. Half-Uttanasana
c. preparation for plank
d. Supported Chaturanga
(with chest on a bolster)
e. downward-facing dog
f. Prasarita Padottanasana
g. forearm plank

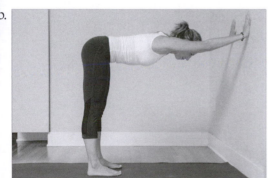

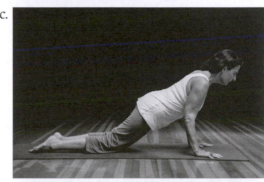

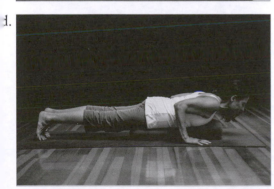

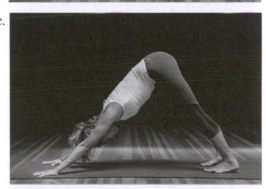

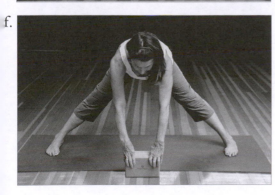

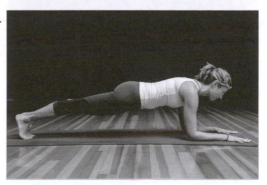

5. Breathing using the diaphragm

Always integrate the proper use of breathing into your class. Begin by having your students lie on their backs and place their hands on their bellies. Teach them to breathe using the main muscle of respiration, the diaphragm. If they are breathing with the diaphragm, the belly should rise on the inhalation and fall on the exhalation. Practicing lying down helps to turn off the neck muscles and makes it much easier to accomplish. Once students are comfortable lying down, they can practice the breathing in a seated position. Then you can begin to integrate the breathing into their asana practice. Explain that proper breathing activates the parasympathetic nervous system, which encourages increased circulation and healing of injured tissues. Also, explain that proper excursion of the diaphragm is essential for normal mobility of the rib cage, which is directly connected to the thoracic vertebrae. If you do not breathe properly, you directly affect the quality of movement of the entire vertebral column. Often, some of my students feel lower back pain as a result of excessive tightness in the upper back. If the upper back is restricted, the lower back has to bear the weight of the world and eventually it will wear out. Postures to practice breathing include: lying on the back with knees bent, lying supine over a bolster, lying over two blocks and sitting in Virasana (hero's pose) on a bolster.

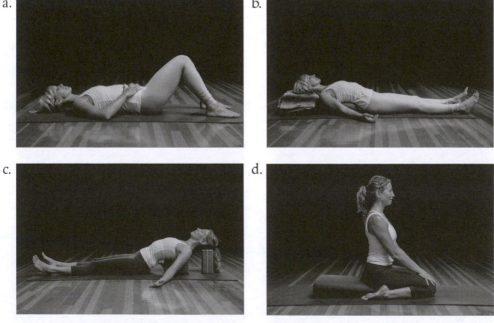

Figure 9.5 Diaphragmatic breathing: a. lying on the back with knees bent; b. lying supine over a bolster; c. lying over two blocks; d. sitting in Virasana on a bolster

6. Postural strengtheners

Work on postural muscles in yoga poses that encourage strength in the smaller muscles of the body. Very often individuals have spent most of their lives strengthening larger muscle groups such as the gluteus maximus and rectus abdominis, instead of the more important, deeper postural muscles like the gluteus medius and the transversus abdominis. Build your students' strength and level of awareness by working with postures that encourage correct activation of deeper muscles related to standing and sitting upright. Encourage subtle strength without tension in Tadasana (mountain pose) and Dandasana (staff pose) variations. Parighasana (gate pose) is an effective posture for your students to work on to lengthen the spine on each side. You can also work on Plank and Side Plank (Vasisthasana) to build the back and core muscles. Standing poses with an emphasis on lifting the pit of the abdomen are also good options for working with postural muscles.

a.
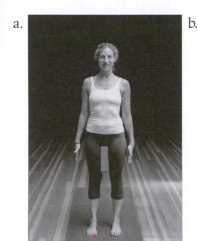
b.
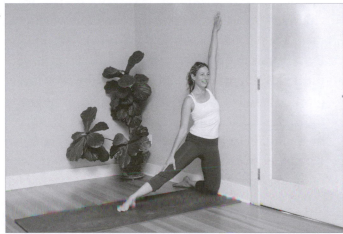

c.
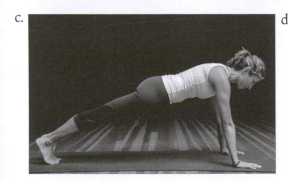
d.
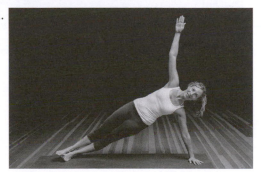

Figure 9.6 Postural muscles sequence: a. Tadasana; b. Parighasana; c. plank; d. side plank (Vasisthasana)

7. Core strengtheners

Teach your students how to maintain the natural curve of the lower back while activating the abdominals, especially the deepest layer, the transversus abdominis. Work on lifting the pit of the abdomen in postures such as mountain pose, supported lunges, gentle back bends, and warrior I in order to encourage length in the spine, both in neutral and in spinal extension. Safe core-strengthening postures can include: plank pose (with knees supported or off the ground), forearm plank, Navasana (boat pose) variations, Jathara Parivartanasana (revolved abdomen pose), and arm lifts on all fours (as illustrated in Chapter 7, Figure 7.10). Make sure that your students learn how to feel when the abdominals are working, as opposed to when the hip flexors are contracting. We all know that we do not need to create more tension in the hip flexors; in most individuals the hip flexors are too tight and often in spasm.

This is a good opportunity to work on ego and competition in the practice. Encourage your students to back off a bit and really feel what is happening. Ask them, "What goes through your mind when you don't go to your limit? Is there a feeling of inadequacy? Of failure? Where does that feeling come from? Do you not feel like you are doing anything if you are not pushing yourself further?" Core strengthening really brings out this egoistic desire in people to push beyond limits. In yoga the abdomen is not meant to be "rock hard." Such tight muscles actually increase tension in the diaphragm and prevent proper breathing. In yoga we are looking for a balance between softness and strength, the ability to call on strength when we need it—not to create a shield or suit of armor around ourselves so that we become hard and push everyone away.

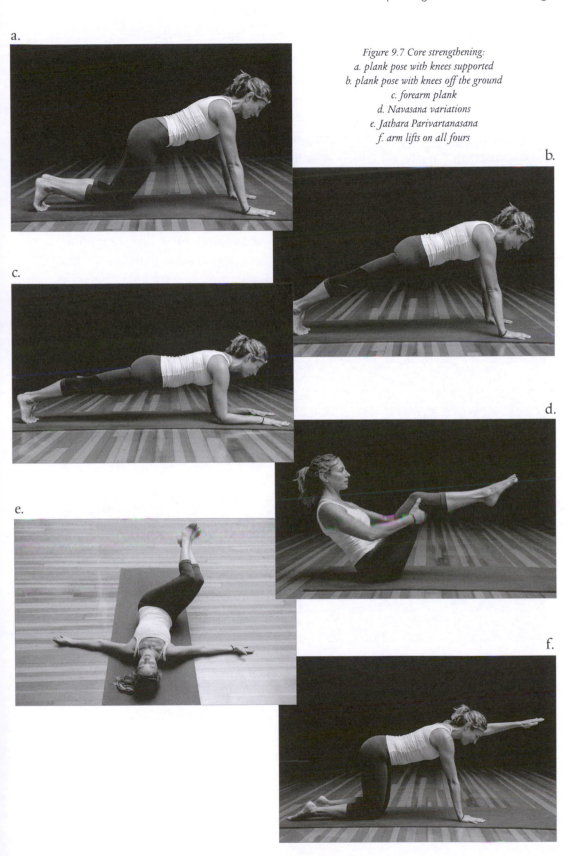

Figure 9.7 Core strengthening:
a. plank pose with knees supported
b. plank pose with knees off the ground
c. forearm plank
d. Navasana variations
e. Jathara Parivartanasana
f. arm lifts on all fours

8. Maintaining length and safety in back bends

In Yoga for a Happy Back it is important to work on reducing fear of back bends. You can explain to your class that back bends are actually safe and encouraged for individuals with back pain. Teach your students that back bends only hurt when we are not aware of maintaining the integrity of the postures. This means that instead of hinging at one level in the spine, as discussed in Chapter 1, which most individuals do during back bends, it is important to maintain length and space between each vertebra, as if the spine were a string of perfectly spaced pearls. If each level is moving into extension, this is indeed healthy for the discs and to balance out a forward head posture and any excessive thoracic kyphosis. Good postures for cultivating spinal extension include: Bhujangasana (cobra), Setu Bandhasana (half-bridge that focuses on lifting the chest and not collapsing in the lower back), Danurasana (bow pose), and Shalabasana (locust).

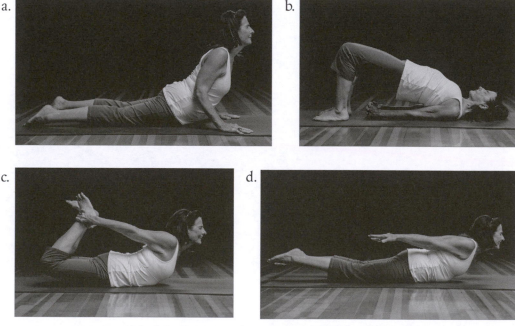

Figure 9.8 Back bends: a. Bhujangasana; b. Setu Bandhasana; c. Danurasana; d. Shalabasana

9. Preparation for forward bends

Even though forward bends are contraindicated for individuals with back pain, I believe that it is important to practice the preparatory work for practicing forward bends safely. Preparation for forward folds includes emphasizing the need to tilt the pelvis anteriorly so as to maintain the lumbar curve, followed by creating a softness in the thoracic spine. These poses are especially helpful for individuals who have decreased thoracic kyphosis (flattened upper back), as it helps to soften and restore the natural curves of the spine. For those with tight hamstrings and the tendency to tip their pelvis backwards into a posterior tilt when sitting, this preparation helps to enhance their ability to move the top of the sacrum into the body before folding forward, again protecting the lower back in all forward bends. Also, the energetics of forward folds is essential for a well-rounded practice, as forward folding encourages the action of going inward and quieting the mind. The sense that the student is left with after this practice is one of tranquility and serenity. Students or clients with anxiety also benefit from practicing forward bends, as they calm the nervous system.

To create a class with an emphasis on forward bends, it is important to open the hamstrings first. Poses to include are: Supta Padangusthasana (reclining hand to big toe pose); Parsva Supta Padangusthasana (side hand to big toe pose); Dandasana (staff pose) sitting on a bolster or folded blanket and emphasizing the anterior pelvic tilt; Ardha Uttanasana (half-standing forward fold); Ardha Parsvottanasana (pyramid pose); Adho Mukha Svanasana (downward-facing dog) maintaining lumbar curve, bending knees as necessary; Upavista Konasana (wide-angled seatedforward bend); Janusirsasana (seated head to knee forward fold); and Paschimottanasana preparation (seated two-legged forward fold) with integrity in the spine. Encourage your students to listen to their bodies and not go beyond their limits, which is when we lose the integrity of our spines. Here, too, you need to encourage them to watch their egos. Have them use a yoga strap as needed around the soles of the feet to keep the spine straight and the sacrum at a minimum of 90° perpendicular to the floor.

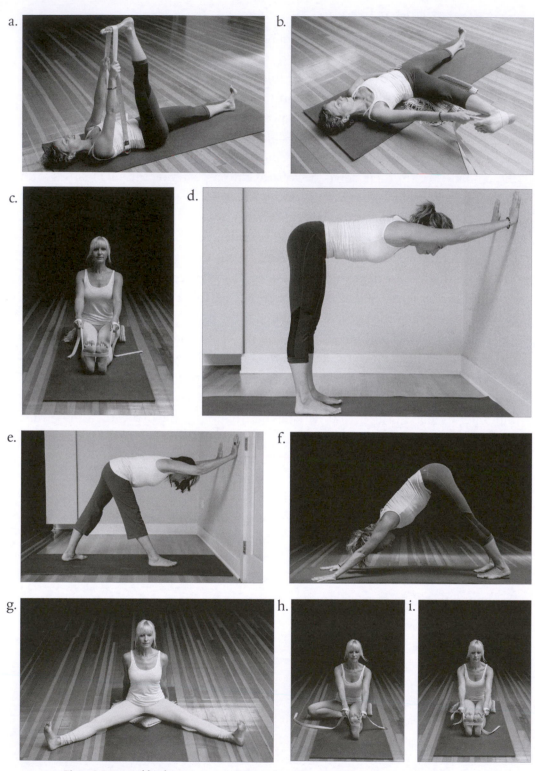

Figure 9.9 *Forward bend preparations: a. Supta Padangusthasana; b. Parsva Supta Padangusthasana; c. Dandasana; d. Ardha uttanasana; e. Ardha Parsvottanasana; f. Adho Mukha Svanasana; g. Upavista Konasana; h. Janusirsasana preparation; i. Paschimottanasana preparation*

10. Safety in twists

Twisting can be very helpful for individuals with back pain, but technique is extremely important in order to preserve spinal health, as the space between each pair of vertebrae decreases naturally as a result of normal biomechanics. Twisting can help heal the spine, as it opens and lengthens muscles that run at a diagonal, such as the obliques and the intercostals. Also, research reported on the naturalheightgrowth.com website (2014) has shown that rotational forces contribute significantly to regeneration of the discs and can actually create some increased height in the disc space as well. The key to twisting safely is to focus on lengthening the spine *before* you twist. Also, it is important to have your students twist from the torso, and not the neck or head. Encourage your students to respect their limitations. If they feel a restriction, they should stop and breathe into it, never forcing in a twist.

Remember, as well, that individuals with scoliosis will likely have more range of motion when twisting to one side than the other, due to the rotational component already present in their spines. Therefore never force anyone, especially someone with scoliosis, into a twist, but rather allow them to lengthen as they inhale and twist on the exhalation, with the intention to open where they are restricted. Twists can also aggravate the SI joint in the event of a sacral torsion; this is because rotation in the spine will cause the sacrum to twist in the opposite direction of movement. For those who suffer from SI joint pain, let the pelvis move as one unit during seated twists as well as standing poses such as Trikonasana (triangle), Parvritta Trikonasana (revolved triangle), and Parsvakonasana (side-angle stretch). If you allow the pelvis to move as one unit, there is less tension on the SI joint, and more rotation is encouraged in the spine instead.

11. Standing poses to strengthen the foundation

I have found that very often "back classes" tend to be equated with "gentle yoga classes." While gentle and restorative yoga is extremely beneficial and should be practiced as part of any regular yoga practice, I also believe that strength is essential for a healthy spine. With this in mind, you will need to work with standing poses in order to build strength in your students' foundation: their legs. The legs support the spine, and when there is weakness in the legs and hip muscles all the weight tends to fall on the joints, including the lumbar spine, pelvis, hips, and knees. If we have strong legs, we can use an essential concept in yoga, which is to focus on "grounding in order to lift." As Newton's Third Law of Motion holds that every action creates an equal and opposite reaction, we all need to press the four corners of the feet into the earth in order to create a response of lifting in the lower belly and lumbar spine. Standing poses are the perfect opportunity to access the strength in the essential postural muscles that support the spine. In addition, they help open the hips in all possible directions. So, don't forget to incorporate strength into your Happy Back classes.

The foundation of all standing poses is found in Tadasana (mountain pose) and therefore it is important to teach this pose first. In my opinion, mastering mountain pose is one of the hardest tasks in all of asana, as there are many instructions and subtleties that require a focused and relaxed mind. Have your students explore Tadasana in many different ways: with their backs against a wall; with a block between the legs (as seen in Chapter 3); with arms elevated; with the palms externally rotated; and with the palms facing the thighs. Guide your students to try mountain pose lying down. How does this change their experience? This is a great option for those who are not so mobile or have challenges with balance.

Some standing poses are especially recommended for sciatica: Trikonasana and Ardha Chandrasana, for instance, both with the front foot externally rotated. This position allows the piriformis muscle to relax and takes pressure off the sciatic nerve. Begin with modified poses focusing on lengthening the spine, opening the hamstrings, and finding a neutral spine, including Half-Uttanasana and Half-Parsvottanasana. Parsvakonasana helps to lengthen the side waist, including the quadratus lumborum muscle, which is hard to lengthen, as well as the obliques and the latissimus dorsi muscle. Modified variations (with block or chair) of Parivrtta Trikonasana open up the rib cage, thoracic spine, and chest, as well as the outer hips and thighs (external rotators of the hip and IT band). Warrior I opens the hip flexors, while warrior III builds strength and stability in the hip extensors and gluteus medius muscle. Prasarita Padottanasana builds leg strength, stretches the adductors, and releases tension in the lower back and SI joint. Warrior II can be a wonderful pose to build strength in the hips and pelvis, as well as open the hips, but tends to aggravate SI joint dysfunction.

For more advanced practitioners Sirsasana (headstand) is an excellent way to strengthen postural muscles; it encourages internal rotation of the thighs and strengthens the serratus anterior muscle and the core. Headstand is essentially Tadasana turned upside down.

For those with acute pain, modified standing poses can be practiced using a wall or horse for support, and a chair.

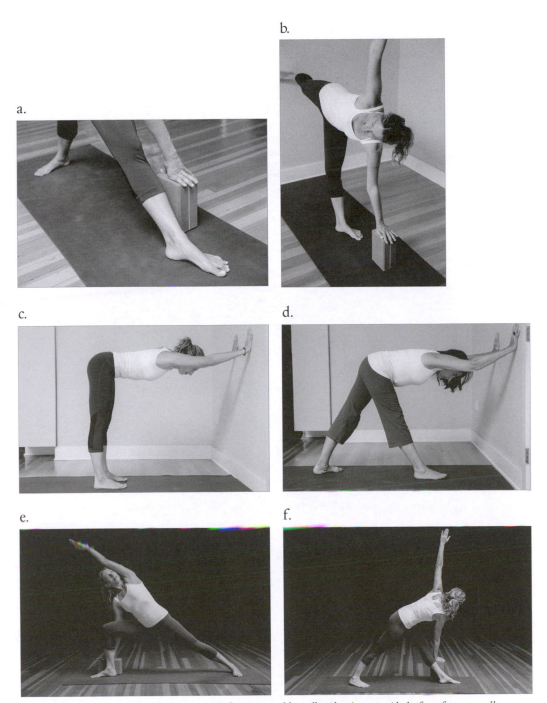

Figure 9.10 Standing pose sequence: a. Trikonasana and b. Ardha Chandrasana with the front foot externally rotated; c. Half Uttanasana; d. Half-Parsvottanasana; e. Parsvakonasana f. Parivrtta Trikonasana;

g.

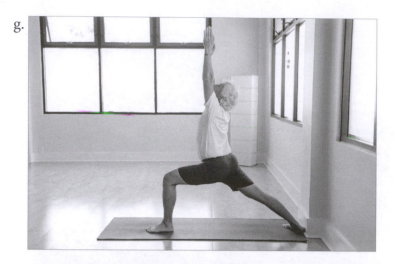

h.

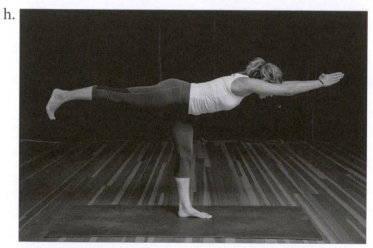

i.

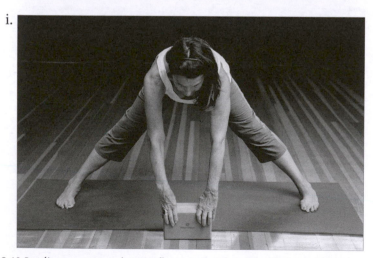

Figure 9.10 Standing pose sequence (continued): g. warrior I; h. warrior III; i. Prasarita Padottanasana

12. Yoga wall and traction

If you are fortunate enough to have access to a yoga wall at home or at your studio, you will discover that a class focusing on traction and hanging on the wall is the most satisfying for those with back pain. The aim of traction is to allow the spinal muscles that clamp down around the vertebrae when there is physical injury or mental/emotional tension to release. This release creates more space between the vertebrae and decreases compression of the nerves, discs, and/or soft tissue. Creating space, as we explored in Chapter 1, is the key to healing from back pain and maintaining a healthy spine.

While traction is heavenly for those with back pain, remember that bilateral traction (traction with both legs) is contraindicated during the acute phase of the injury. Move slowly with your students and make sure that they do not have an adverse reaction when they come out of traction. Do multiple repetitions with shorter holds before hanging for a long period of time. Get the body used to the idea of letting go and trusting that it can release its grip on the spine, and all will be well. Start with unilateral traction, bending one knee at a time in Adho Mukha Svanasana on wall ropes. Start with supine unilateral traction (as illustrated in Chapter 3) and the low back series. Then move into the inversions recommended in Chapter 6. The two best poses to practice regularly are Adho Mukha Svanasana and hanging traction. I often recommend that individuals, especially those with scoliosis, buy a wall for home use and hang for a few minutes each day. Besides the lengthening effects on the spine, the powerful calming effects of inversions are a welcome bonus.

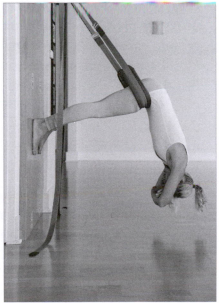

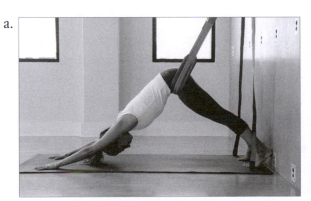

Figure 9.11 a. Adho Mukha Svanasana;
b. hanging traction on yoga wall

When you ask your students to hang from the wall, instruct them to use their breath and awareness to release tension in the spine. Have them think about the side waist lengthening and the pelvis and rib cage moving in opposite directions.

If you do not have a yoga wall, you can guide them to practice partner poses that mimic the effects of the wall ropes. Have students pull in pairs in downward-facing dog, or in threes in Ardha Parsvottanasana. Give them a sense of what the poses can feel like with a yoga strap in the hip crease. Then teach them to engage their quadriceps and deepen the hip crease/groin area in order to create their own sense of traction.

a.
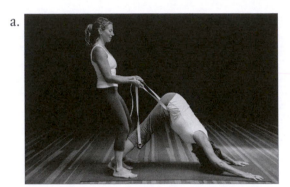

b.
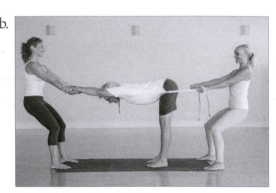

Figure 9.12 Partner poses for traction: a. Adho Mukha Svanasana in pairs;
b. Ardha Parsvottanasana and Ardha Uttanasana in threes

13. Chest openers, chest openers, chest openers!

Let's face it: most of us spend our lives bent forward, leaning over a desk or sitting slumped forward at a computer. Everyone benefits from chest openers, as they encourage a proper posture for standing, walking, and breathing. Most back pain can be corrected simply by opening the chest and the hips so that there is a better distribution of weight throughout the natural curves of the spine, and a better posture when standing, sitting, and walking. Opening the chest also allows for a better excursion of the diaphragm, and better thoracic mobility. It is also preparation for meditation and pranayama, which is the aim of asana practice in the first place.

You can see from this list of themes that there are plenty of options available when creating classes for a Happy Back. There may be some individuals who cannot accomplish everything, but with your knowledge of different conditions and modifications you should be able to adapt accordingly. Teaching Yoga for a Happy Back will require you to be able to find modifications for students who are more limited than others quickly and spontaneously, so it is important to practice these techniques and refine them as much as possible at home and in private sessions.

Then it will be up to you to add another layer to your classes by integrating yoga philosophy and the five koshas into the classes so that your students can understand how yoga facilitates healing or, at the very least, lessens suffering and increases well-being.

Themes integrating yoga philosophy

1. Balancing effort and ease

Design a class in which all the poses are practiced with a balance of effort and ease. Read the yoga sutra to your students, *Sthira sukham asanam* ("The poses in yoga should be steady and comfortable"), and explain that this is one of the only sutras that talks about asana, the physical practice of yoga. Let them know that the yoga sutras place more emphasis on the spiritual and meditative aspects of yoga, and that the physical poses are simply there to support their evolution and transformation; they are not an end in themselves. The beauty of this sutra is that it gives us a prescription for how to practice not only the poses, but also everything in life. We can learn how to work hard without increasing unnecessary tension in the body. We can learn that effort does not mean "gripping" or "pushing" beyond boundaries to satisfy the ego's desire to "be the best" or to "be good enough." We can learn that yoga is the practice of finding balance and comfort in poses that require physical effort, but equally that we need to be vigilant and awake and focused during relaxing and restorative postures as well.

2. Grounding in order to lift

This is an important concept to illustrate in all poses (especially standing poses and inversions), as well as for correct posture and gait. Yoga is about contradiction. We push the weight into all four corners of the feet so that we can lift the insteps and the spine in Tadasana (mountain pose). We push into the index finger mound in order to lengthen the chest, sides of the waist, and pelvis in downward-facing dog. We push the big toe mound of the front leg into the earth as we draw the outer hip backwards in Parsvottanasana (pyramid pose) in order to keep the pelvis level and open the outer hips. This concept is everywhere in asana as well as in spiritual aspiration. In order to lift ourselves up to a higher level, we need to focus on rooting ourselves on this earth. Trees need to grow roots in order to get taller. If they grow but do not have deep roots, they will fall. So, emphasize to your students that they should focus on rooting down in all their poses, and on their connection to the earth. Explain to them that, with this intention, they will cultivate more calmness, presence, and stability while also reaching for new heights.

3. Bringing the mind into the body

Incorporate this theme into your classes in order to teach your students how yoga actually works to heal. The difference between yoga and other forms of physical activity is the attention, awareness, and intention that we put into the postures. By focusing the mind on the instructions and subtle actions of the body, we bring the mind into the body as a form of meditation. Our mind is then given a break from its usual state of flying about in a million different directions, and instead can practice one-pointed focus—the sixth "limb" of yoga known as Dharana. Over time, while increasing awareness and control of the body as a great side effect, your students will experience the main benefit of their practice: a mind that is more calm and focused.

The second of the *Yoga Sutras of Patanjali* teaches: *yoga chitta vritti nirodha*. The Ashtanga Yoga website translates this to read: "When you are in a state of yoga, all misconceptions (*vrittis*) that can exist in the mutable aspect of human beings (*chitta*) disappear." In other words, a regular yoga practice will still the fluctuations of the mind and quiet any changes of mood. In the context of yoga, the presence of vrittis (fluctuations) in consciousness is regarded as an impediment to enlightenment. In his often quoted *Raja Yoga*, the nineteenth-century sage Swami Vivekananda uses the metaphor of a lake to illustrate these disturbances in consciousness, with chitta as the mind stuff and vrittis as the waves and ripples rising to the surface when external causes affect it. It is only possible to see to the bottom when the ripples have subsided, and the water is calm, clear, and transparent. If the water is muddy it will also obscure the bottom.

As you teach your Happy Back classes, remind your students of this wisdom: the bottom of the lake is their true Self, peaceful and free. Pain in the body is often exacerbated and magnified by mental and emotional tension, so encourage them to work on the mind as an integral part of the healing process, instead of masking the discomfort with medication and other tools of distraction. Have your students pay attention to those moments in class when their minds wander; keep encouraging them to come back to the breath and the actions of the various parts of their bodies.

4. Integrity

Integrity is one of my favorite topics to explore in a class setting. Within the context of this theme, I like to work with alignment in all postures and stabilization and strengthening during all of the standing and seated poses. Focusing on integrity means watching your students' alignment, slowing down, taming the ego, and respecting the teacher. This class theme is especially important for individuals with SI joint dysfunction, as their main objective is to build strength and stability in the pelvis and surrounding joints. The main focus in this class would be poses with a closed pelvis, meaning both frontal hip bones are pointing straight ahead, as well as strengthening the inner thighs (adductors), pelvic floor musculature, and deep abdominals (transversus abdominis).

When working with integrity it is important to emphasize the difference between strength and stability in the postures, as opposed to hardness or gripping. All too often we approach our yoga practice as we do the rest of our lives. Sometimes we take on an extra challenge or another opportunity to compete with others or with ourselves. Watch any tendency in your students to do the poses with too much of the zealousness that can make the muscles become hard and tense. There is a difference between being strong, steady, and relaxed and being strong and tight or tense from forcing or "overworking" muscles. The first approach is sustainable and peaceful; the other approach is the complete opposite. Sometimes your students may develop injuries because they push too hard. Explain to them that yoga teaches us to look at such tendencies and to find balance. If you see students who are overly competitive, guide them to relax in some of the strengthening poses. If you see others who have the tendency to be lazy and have difficulty working hard in the postures, then encourage them to develop a practice in which they work a bit more vigorously and with complete focus during their time on the mat.

5. Yamas and Niyamas

When designing your class series, another effective organizational idea is to teach students about the Yamas and Niyamas by choosing one each week to focus on and integrate it into your classes. For example, *Ahimsa*, translated as "non-harming," can be taught in the context of noticing if you are practicing your asana in a way that may be harmful for you and your body. Ask your students: how can they practice non-harming if they are not compassionate towards themselves both on and off the mat? Another example is *Satya* (or Truthfulness), which can be practiced in class by teaching people to connect with their own deepest Truth. They should know how far to go, as well as when it is too much, and respect their limitations. Encourage your students to tap into the Heart Center (Anahata Chakra) throughout their practice and to connect with their heart's longing. When they can access their individual Truths, the voices that tell them what they "should" do can be quieted and their true Self can be revealed. Once this is apparent, even if only for a brief moment, your student will know exactly how much asana to practice and what he or she needs on any given day.

As a teacher your role is to help your students find this inner truth, not to serve your own egoistic needs, nor to help push them further towards theirs. We are here to help them find their truth, which is different from our truth. In the *Upanishads*, as translated by Swami Sivananda (1993), the Vedanta Sara Upanishad, Mantra 3, says: "The Self is hidden in all beings like butter in milk." Teach your students that their consistent practice with clear intention is the "churning" that is needed to help them transform.

6. Themes from *Fire of Love*

Probably my favorite way to find inspiration for my classes lies in returning to my teacher Aadil Palkhivala's book, *Fire of Love* (Palkhivala 2008a). I find that the more I read it, the more I discover about myself, about yoga, and about life in general. Very often I will use the book as a reference (after reading through it a few times, of course) and choose one of the themes that my teacher offers so beautifully to design my class. I may choose a saying, story, or quote from any one chapter, and structure my class around that theme. The themes that Aadil presents (in order) are: Dharma, Truth, Integrity, Feeling, Respect, Balance, Bliss, Peace, and Love. Work with any and all of these themes in a Yoga for a Happy Back class. Essentially, if you teach your students how to find their own personal Dharma (purpose or life's mission) and to live it fully, they will no longer experience the same pain and suffering.

As Aadil writes in *Fire of Love* (p.33): "As we evolve, our asana practice remains important, but if we focus entirely on it and make the performance of the poses the end of the endeavor, our practice becomes an obstacle to our own evolution. Asana is to be done not for the sake of asana, but for the sake of dharma."

Determining where to go with the class

Once you have your physical and/or philosophical theme, you must next decide how you are going to design the class and build a sequence of postures that support the theme. I tend to design classes based on three formats.

1. Focus on a marker pose

In this model you will have one pose in mind that you want to build up to. In order to allow your students to accomplish this pose, you will need to choose beginning poses that open and strengthen the muscles that are needed in order to accomplish this pose safely. You can choose your marker pose and then construct a class based on a series of postures that prepare for the pose, practice the marker pose in various ways, and then construct a sequence to help the body unwind from that pose, incorporating appropriate spinal releases. For example, you can choose a pose such as Virabhadrasana I (warrior I) as your marker pose. In order to accomplish this posture and achieve more freedom in the lower back, it is important to open the hip flexors so that they do not pull the lumbar spine into extension (as seen in Chapter 2, Figure 2.4 a.) and create more compression in this pose. It is also important to open the chest and shoulders as well as the rib cage and sides of the waist, in order to achieve more length in the spine. You can now build your sequence around teaching these principles to your students. Practice chest openers in the beginning like Gomukhasana (cowface pose) and Parvatasana (seated cross-legged mountain pose, arms lifted overhead). Encourage length in the spine in Uttitha Balasana (extended child's pose) and in Adho Mukha Svanasana (downward-facing dog). Work on lifting the arms overhead without tensing the neck muscles and maintaining a lift in the POA in Tadasana so that these instructions can be brought into Virabhadrasana I (warrior I). Practice creating length in the lower back during spinal extension in Bhujangasana (cobra pose) or preparations for this pose. To open the hip flexors, practice supported lunges, lunges with the back leg up the wall, Eka Pada Supta Virasana (one-legged reclining hero's pose), and variations from the hip opening series outlined in Chapter 4. You can also prepare for warrior I by practicing twists such as Parivrtta Trikonasana (revolved triangle pose) and/or seated twists. Twists help to open up the intercostal muscles, as they lie at an angle between the ribs. Once they are stretched in twists, there is more space between the ribs available for back bends, the result being less compression in the lower back.

After this warm-up, take the student into different variations of the pose in order to increase their awareness of the subtleties required to practice this asana safely. You can begin with your heel off the ground (which helps keep the pelvis square), and then with the hands at the wall (to encourage extension in the upper back and the proper use of the serratus anterior muscles, and to strengthen the legs). You can also have your students place a thin block, an inclined board, or a blanket under their back heel to give them a sense of grounding and pushing the heel into the earth as an anchor for the posture.

Use a chair to support the front thigh and to encourage more lift in the belly. When they are finally prepared to come into the full pose, we want them to experience freedom in the lumbar spine and length (even stretching) in the front body.

After practicing the variations and culminating in the full posture with all this new awareness, then you can introduce spinal releases to calm the lower back down, in case it is not accustomed to extension exercises. Good releases include: Adho Mukha Svanasana (downward-facing dog); Ardha Uttanasana (half or full forward fold); Prasarita Padottanasana (wide-legged forward fold); Parsva Prasarita Padottanasana (revolved wide-legged forward fold); Upavista Konasana (seated wide-legged forward fold); Parsva Upavista Konasana (revolved seated wide-legged forward fold); Supta Eka Pada Rajakapotasana (reclining one-legged king pigeon pose); a supine spinal twist; and knees to chest. Hanging traction on the wall rope system would also be very beneficial after working on this posture. In Savasana, have your students become aware of the opening in the hip flexors and chest area, inviting breath into those areas and releasing tension on the exhalation.

Using this model, you can help your students achieve a new level of awareness in a specific posture or set of postures, as well as increase their understanding of the instructions required to go deeper and feel freedom in more challenging poses.

2. Focus on certain muscle groups or ranges of motion and go deeper

Using your knowledge of anatomy and biomechanics, you can construct a class that focuses on a group of postures that accomplish a similar result. You can teach a class emphasizing hip openers, chest openers, psoas openers, awareness of the descent and spreading of the shoulder blades, or creating length in the lower back, to name a few. Choose one theme and then pick the best poses that illustrate the theme, and allow your students to experience the results.

Teaching in this fashion will allow your students to leave with a solid understanding of one or more concepts that are integral to their yoga practice and how these themes can be woven throughout many different poses.

3. Make a monthly schedule

One thing I particularly enjoy about certain Iyengar teachers is that such teachers often structure the practice on a monthly basis. The first week of the month is standing poses, followed by forward bends in Week 2, back bends in Week 3, and inversions and/or restoratives in the last week of the month. Using this model, you can be sure that your students will benefit from all the different postures and have a well-rounded practice (assuming they come each week). It also gives them a focus on what to work on at home and can give you more consistency in your teaching. The only caveat here is that the week at hand may not be the best choice for your students that day, depending on what is going on in their life, and also, depending on their Ayurvedic constitution. So when using this kind of schedule, make sure to pay close attention and teach your students to check in with themselves about what they need each day. This will be difficult for beginners to do, as beginners will not have the subtle self-awareness necessary to know what is best for them. Give beginners more structure and teach them how to become more self-referential and grow more sensitive. For your intermediate and advanced students, give them the option to know what they need and practice accordingly, which may include backing off. They can elect to practice a restorative sequence on days where the class may be too intense or active for an individual. Teach your students to listen to their inner voices.

In essence, your students should feel calmer, and more balanced, energized, and focused at the end of a class. They should be more connected to their Heart Center and more embodied overall. In one of Judith Hanson Lasater's workshops that I attended, she recommended asking your students, "What is the residue of the pose?" I love this. Instead of moving quickly through postures with an achievement-oriented approach, encourage your students to make their practice one of self-exploration and continuous curiosity. Teach them to use yoga as a process of investigation and to become more sensitive each day.

Ultimately, an intelligent and effective class creates a mutual relationship and responsibility between the teacher and student. As a teacher, it is your responsibility to create wise and logical classes with accurate instructions tailored to your students' needs. Encourage your students to take responsibility for listening to their bodies' messages and knowing when to work harder and when to slow down. For both teacher and student, an effective class becomes a dance of listening, feeling, and letting go, as well as a process of transformation through awareness and presence.

CHAPTER 10

Sequences to Treat Specific Conditions

Teach people, not poses.
Aadil Palkhivala

Yoga therapy differs from the traditional medical model in several ways, the most significant of which is that a yoga therapist may treat two individuals with the same condition by prescribing completely different physical asana programs and meditation and pranayama techniques due to their very different needs from the perspective of the kosha model. With this in mind, it is difficult and, often, quite limiting to list prescriptions of asana for various conditions because that reduces our work to the most superficial layer, *annamaya kosha*, the physical sheath. Nevertheless, it is important to have a place to begin, a reference point from which we can grow our work into deeper and more intuitive transformative healing. That is the intention of this chapter—not to give you a set of exercises to use for each patient with the same particular condition, but rather to provide a map that will orient you and your client to the beginning of the journey, as well as some suggestions for safe postures that can benefit and heal the physical body. This map should provide you with a place from which to explore and expand as you accumulate more experience in the field. It also offers an opportunity for you to do the practices below and see how they feel in *your* body. I recommend that you practice all of the asanas for a minimum of six months before teaching the postures to others. Unless you have embodied these postures, you cannot transmit the effects to your students.

Most lower back pain falls into one of two categories: *mechanical back pain* or *compressive back pain*. Mechanical back pain refers to any injury or inflammation that is related to the discs, facets, ligaments, muscles, and/or soft tissue around the spine. In these cases the pain is a result of strain or dysfunction that is related to the way that the individual moves, or due to poor posture. Trauma can also cause a disruption to the same structures listed above, and thus create mechanical back pain. Injuries that fall into this category include wear and tear on the discs and joints of the vertebrae (arthritis), muscle strains, ligamentous injuries, and fractures of the vertebrae.

Compressive pain involves pressure or pinching on the spinal nerves or the spinal cord itself and presents with neurological symptoms including tingling, numbness, weakness in the lower extremities, and pain radiating down the buttocks and back of the thigh and calf. Nerve pain is usually caused by a bulging or herniated disc, but can also be due to compression of the nerve in the intervertebral space as it exits the spinal cord.

It is important for you to distinguish between the two types of back pain, as the method of treatment differs for each. In the case of mechanical back pain, we want to address the dysfunction that is causing the pain and provide exercises that encourage proper posture and spinal mobility. For compressive pain, we need to focus on decompression techniques and *creating space* (as mentioned in Chapter 1) between the vertebrae, so that the nerve is not compromised. The main technique for this is *traction*, coupled with intelligent exercises, to reduce the likelihood of continued compressive forces.

In both cases, it is not enough simply to treat the inflammation with medication and/or steroid injections. Those often-used techniques help with the pain temporarily by treating the symptoms, but they do not treat the source of the problem. *Long-term healing only occurs when we look at the origin of the pain and make corrections that impact the biomechanics of the spine.* If this is ignored, your student will experience recurrent bouts of the same problem on a regular basis. This chapter offers you safe, effective yoga sequences to share with students and clients to gradually heal both kinds of back pain.

The following sequences are meant as a guideline only. Remember to teach your students, and not just the poses. Use your professional judgment, and do modify or omit any of the poses listed according to your students' needs and abilities.

1. DEGENERATIVE DISC DISEASE OR ARTHRITIS

Degenerative disc disease (DDD) is one of the most common causes of lower back and neck pain. The terms "degeneration" and "disease" often cause alarm for those who receive this diagnosis. The truth of the matter is that DDD essentially means the same thing as arthritis; it refers to the wearing down of the discs of the spine due to normal use and/or aging. It is not, in fact, a progressive disease at all, but is simply a function of normal life and the effect of gravity on the spine. Many individuals have DDD and do not experience any symptoms at all. It is for this reason that we should evaluate where there is tightness and weakness in the body and investigate the cause of pain further. Explain to your clients that most individuals have DDD

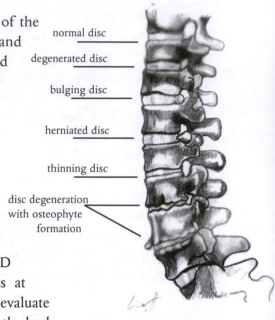

normal disc

degenerated disc

bulging disc

herniated disc

thinning disc

disc degeneration with osteophyte formation

Figure 10.1 Degenerative disc disease of the lumbar spine/arthritis

but not all of them have pain associated with it. Ease their fears about having an "unstable" spine and let them know that there are no restrictions other than their own pain during their yoga practice. Yoga is helpful for individuals with arthritis and DDD as it encourages length in the muscles of the spine and pelvis. The more we stretch and remain supple with an emphasis on length in the spine, the less compression there will be between the joints of the vertebrae. As long as there is no rubbing of one joint on the other, there is no pain.

Yoga asana for this condition should include hip openers to create optimal pelvic alignment and encourage a natural lumbar curve. There should also be an emphasis on postures that create length in the spine, including traction and chest openers to open up the rib cage and anterior chest musculature. Finally, you should instruct your client in the correct methods to strengthen the spinal extensors, abdominals, and pelvic floor to encourage stability during activities of daily living. The Purna Yoga Reversing the Aging of the Spine Series in Chapter 6 is especially recommended for those with DDD, as it encourages mobility in the spine *with traction*.

DEGENERATIVE DISC DISEASE/ARTHRITIS

Recommendations

- Purna Yoga Hip Opening Series
- Purna Yoga Reversing the Aging of the Spine Series
- Chest openers
- Back strengtheners
- Abdominal strengtheners

Contraindications

- None; practice as tolerated

Degenerative disc disease sequence

a. Purna Yoga Hip Opening Series (see Chapter 4)

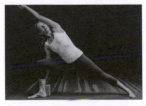

b. Yoga Mudra (straight ahead and walking hands to the side)

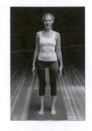

c. Supported lunge

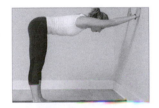

d. Half-Uttanasana (half forward fold) at wall

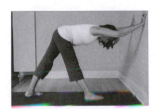

e. Half-Parsvottanasana at the wall (half-pyramid pose at wall)

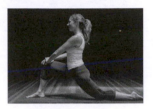

f. Tadasana with block

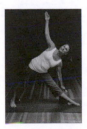

g. Trikonasana (triangle pose)

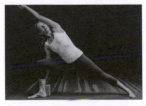

h. Parsvakonasana (extended side angle pose)

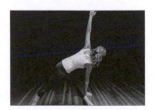

i. Parivrtta Trikonasana revolved triangle pose with chair or blocks as needed

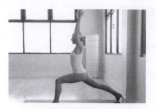

j. Virabhadrasana I (warrior I)

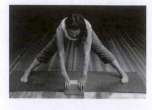

k. Prasarita Padottanasana (wide-legged standing forward bend)

l. Purna Yoga Reversing the Aging of the Spine Series (see Chapter 6)

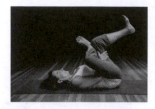

m. Supta Eka Pada Rajakapotasana (supine pigeon)

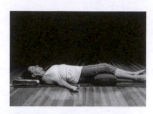

n. Savasana (corpse pose) with feet on bolster or chair

2. FACET JOINT SYNDROME

As illustrated in Chapter 2, the facet joints are the joints in which movement occurs in the spine in all directions. One of the most common causes of lower back pain is compression between the surfaces of the superior and inferior facets at one or more levels, a condition that causes inflammation, and therefore pain. As both surfaces are lined with cartilage and bathed in synovial fluid, if there is damage to the cartilage or to the integrity of the joint, there will be painful rubbing of bone on bone. With facet joint syndrome there is no nerve root involvement, and

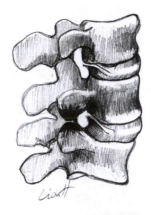

Figure 10.2 Facet joint syndrome

therefore no neurological signs and symptoms. Part of treating this may require an evaluation by a licensed physical therapist to evaluate whether there is a positional or motion dysfunction so they can adjust the spine accordingly. From a yoga perspective, the goal is to create as much traction and length as possible between each pair of vertebrae and to open up the hips and surrounding spinal musculature so that there is maximum space between the two joint surfaces on the facets.

FACET JOINT SYNDROME

Recommendations

- Poses that encourage proper alignment in the spinal column
- Spinal traction
- Hip opening

Contraindications

- None; practice as tolerated
- Never force someone with scoliosis into a deep twist, especially on the side that is more limited, as this can cause compression of facet joints

Facet joint syndrome sequence

a. Purna Yoga Low Back Series
(see Chapter 3)

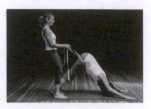
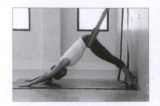

b. Adho Mukha Svanasana (downward-facing dog) on
yoga wall, or with partner, using a strap

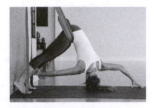
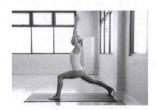
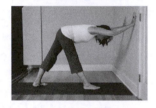

c. Cross stretch and twist on yoga wall d. Half-Uttanasana (half forward fold)

e. Trikonasana (triangle pose)

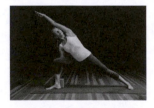
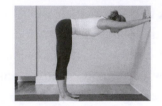

f. Parsvakonasana (extended
side angle pose)

g. Virabhadrasana I (warrior I)

h. Half-Parsvottanasana
(half-pyramid pose)

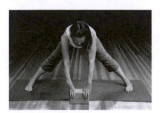
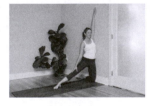
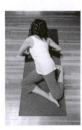

i. Prasarita Padottanasana (extended
separate leg stretching pose)

j. Parighasana (gate pose)
against a wall

k. Matsyangasana (mermaid's pose)

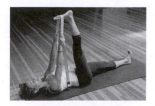

l. Supta Padangusthasana
(hamstring stretch)

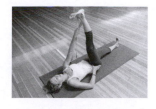

m. Parivrtta Supta Padangusthasana
(outer hip stretch)

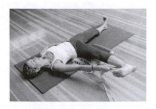

n. Parsva Supta Padangusthasana
(inner thigh stretch in side-
reclined big toe pose)

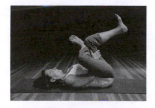

o. Piriformis stretch

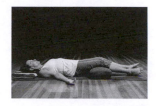

p. Savasana (corpse pose)

3. SCOLIOSIS

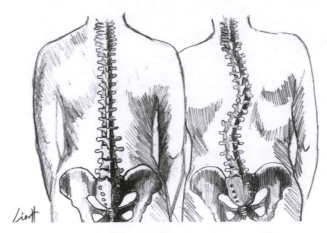

Figure 10.3 Scoliosis

Scoliosis is a condition in which three or more vertebrae are laterally flexed to one side and rotated to the opposite side. It looks like an S-shaped curve from the back, as there is usually a compensatory curve above and below the primary area. Scoliosis often occurs in young girls aged 10–16, during their growth spurt. In most cases the cause is unknown (idiopathic) and does not progress into adulthood. According to the WebMD website, "Approximately 2 percent to 3 percent of Americans at age 16 have scoliosis. Less than 0.1 percent have spinal curves measuring greater than 40°, which is the point at which surgery becomes a consideration."

Although most cases of scoliosis are mild, there are consequences that play out in activities of daily living, especially in yoga practice. Because there is a C-shaped curve, the muscles on the concave side of the spine are shortened and tight, while the convex side of the curve is overstretched and weak. If the curve is concave to the left (as in Figure 10.3), the spine will also be rotated to the right, since in scoliosis the rotational component is always opposite to the side of the curvature. Because the vertebrae are side bent and slightly rotated, there is an increased chance of compression between the facet joints, as well as degeneration and disc protrusions. The aim of yoga for scoliosis is to create length and symmetry as best as possible, to lengthen the shortened side of the curve and to strengthen the lengthened side of the curve, thereby decreasing the curvature or, at the very least, stopping it from progressing with time.

It is also important to remember to practice gently, so that you do not force the spine into any ranges of motion that may be biomechanically limited. When practiced with mindfulness and awareness, yoga can help those with scoliosis avoid back pain or, with a steady discipline and focused work with a teacher, can even correct a great deal of the curvature.

A complete, well-rounded yoga practice would benefit all individuals with scoliosis, as the emphasis of most postures is length and openness of the rib cage, chest, and lumbar spine, as well as optimal activation of the diaphragm for effective breathing. In order to correct the curvature, postures that emphasize lengthening the shortened side and strengthening the lengthened side should be encouraged. Symmetry and length should also be emphasized for students with scoliosis. I go into greater detail about scoliosis and yoga-based treatments for the condition in my upcoming book *Scoliosis: Yoga Therapy and the Art of Letting Go.*

SCOLIOSIS

Recommendations

- Poses to create length in the spine
- Spinal traction
- Hip openers
- Supported positions with assistance to counteract curvature
- Gentle chest openers
- Vasisthasana (side plank) on convex side of curve

Contraindications

- None; avoid pain and be careful during twists, especially on the limited side

Scoliosis sequence

a. *Purna Yoga Hip Opening Series (see Chapter 4)*

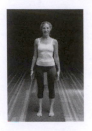

b. *Tadasana (mountain pose) with block, emphasizing equal weight in both feet*

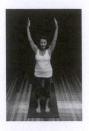

c. *Utthita Tadasana (arms overhead) to increase length and strength of the trunk without overarching the back or shifting the hips anteriorly*

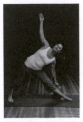

d. *Trikonasana (triangle pose) with yoga wall to help keep space between lower ribs and pelvis*

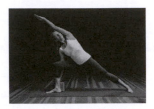

e. *Parsvakonasana (extended side angle pose)—more often on concave (shortened) side of the curve*

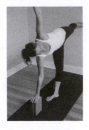

f. *Ardha Chandrasana (half-moon pose) with foot on wall*

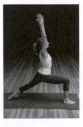

g. *Virabhadrasana I (warrior I) with arms extended to open chest*

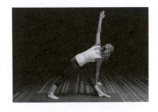

h. *Parivrtta Trikonasana (triangle pose)*

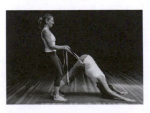

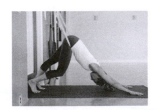

i. *Adho Mukha Svanasana (downward-facing dog) on wall ropes or with a partner; work on lengthening short side of the trunk*

j. *Cross stretch on wall ropes*

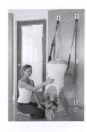

k. Hanging traction; moving breath throughout the spine

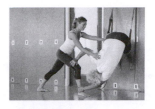

l. Purna Yoga Reversing the Aging of the Spine Series (especially lateral flexion to lengthen concave side of the curve)

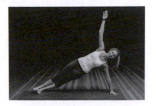

m. Vasisthasana (side plank) (to build side muscles) on the convex side of the curve

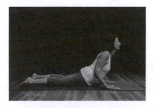

n. Bhujangasana (cobra pose)

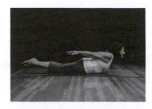

o. Salabhasana (locust pose)

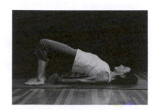

p. Setu Bandha Sarvangasana (bridge pose)

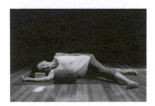

q. Side lying over a towel roll under the apex of the curve on the convex side

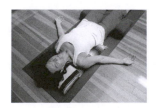

r. Savasana (corpse pose) with support under lower side

4. STENOSIS

Stenosis is an abnormal narrowing of the spinal canal that can create pressure on the spinal cord. Generally, spinal extension decreases the diameter of the spinal canal, the area where the spinal cord is situated; therefore individuals usually feel discomfort in extension, and

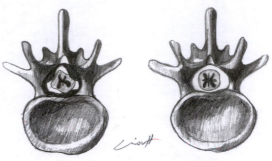

Figure 10.4 Stenosis

relief from symptoms when they bend forward. It is for this reason that spinal extension exercises (back bending postures) are contraindicated for those with spinal stenosis. In the physical practice of yoga it is important to focus on opening the hips, and doing postural exercises to maintain the natural spinal curves and to strengthen the back in neutral. Abdominal and pelvic floor strengthening is encouraged as well, to increase spinal and pelvic stability.

SPINAL STENOSIS

Recommendations

- Poses to work on length in the spine
- Core strengthening in neutral/ slight lumbar flexion
- Hip openers
- Chest openers
- Back bend preparation in neutral, e.g. Bhujangasana (cobra pose) with the forehead on the floor—without coming up into full extension

Contraindications

- All back bends beyond neutral position

Stenosis sequence

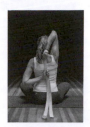

a. Gomukhasana arms (cowface arms)

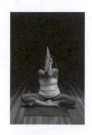

b. Garudasana arms (eagle arms)

c. Purna Yoga Hip Opening Series (see Chapter 4)

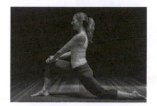

d. Supported lunge

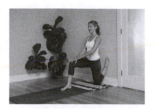

e. Lunge with leg up wall—to open quads and psoas further

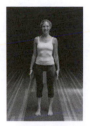

f. Tadasana (mountain pose) with block

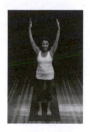

g. Utthita Tadasana (extended mountain pose)

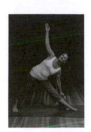

h. Trikonasana (triangle pose)

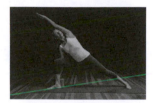

i. Parsvakonasana (extended side angle pose)

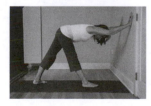

j. Half-Parsvottanasana (half-pyramid pose)

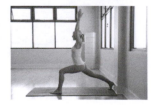

k. Virabhadrasana I (warrior I)

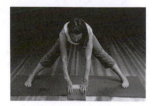

l. Prasarita Padottanasana (wide-legged forward fold)

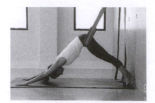 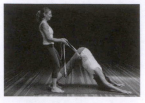 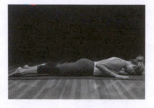

m. Adho Mukha Svanasana (downward-facing dog) on wall ropes or with partner

n. Marichyasana I (sage pose)

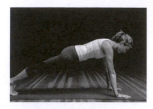 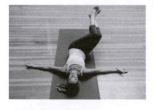

o. Phalakasana (plank pose)

p. Modified Bhujangasana (cobra pose) with forehead on the floor (no spinal extension)—focus on lengthening the spine by pulling hands back towards your hips and bringing the rib cage forward towards the front of the mat

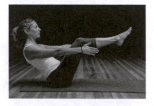 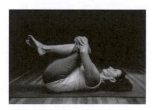 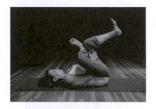

q. Navasana (boat pose) variations

r. Jathara Parivartanasana (revolved abdomen pose)

s. Supine piriformis stretch

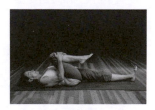 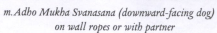 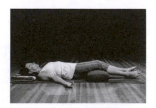

t. Half-Apanasana (single knee to chest)

u. Apanasana (double knees to chest)

v. Savasana (corpse pose) with legs over bolster

5. SPONDYLOLISTHESIS

Spondylolisthesis is a condition in which there is a fracture in a part of the vertebra called the pars interarticularis (see Figure 10.5). This break in the vertebra causes one vertebra to slide forward over the one below it. This anterior displacement of one vertebra can cause pinching on the nerves or spinal cord, although sometimes no symptoms are present at all. Spondylolisthesis can be congenital (present at birth) or can develop from overuse, trauma, infection, or arthritis. It is often present in teens and young adults who participate in sports such as gymnastics and weight lifting—activities that place excessive force

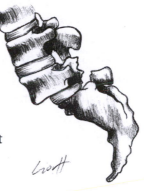

Figure 10.5 Spondylolisthesis

on the vertebrae. Because one of the vertebrae slides forward on the other, spinal extension postures (back bends) are contraindicated in individuals with spondylolisthesis. Their yoga practice is similar to that for those with stenosis, and should focus on creating space in the spine, normalizing the curves, keeping the chest and hips open, and strengthening the core and back muscles in a neutral position.

SPONDYLOLISTHESIS

Recommendations

- Poses to work on length in the spine
- Core strengthening in neutral/ slight lumbar flexion
- Hip openers
- Chest openers
- Back bend preparation in neutral

Contraindications

- All back bends beyond neutral position

Spondylolisthesis sequence

Same as stenosis sequence above.

6. SACROILIAC JOINT DYSFUNCTION

As we discussed in detail in Chapter 5, pain in the sacroiliac (SI) region is usually caused by abnormal movement in the SI joint—either too much or too little—which typically results in inflammation and pain. Trauma and overuse can also cause pain and dysfunction in this joint, and there tends to be an increase in symptoms in yoga practitioners who are overly flexible. The SI joint is a joint of stability; overstretching of ligaments in this area, sometimes due to overdoing seated forward bends and twists, can exacerbate the problem. Yoga asana (the physical practice) will not help to realign a sacrum that is experiencing

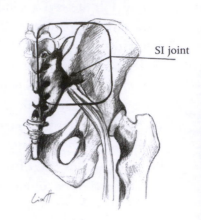

SI joint

Figure 10.6 sacroiliac joint dysfunction

a torsion or rotational force, and it is important to seek professional help for realignment. Once the sacrum is back in place, the student will be able to go back to a regular practice, but may want to modify certain poses that create strain on the SI joint. They will need to focus more on strengthening the hip, abdominals, and pelvic floor muscles and decreasing their need to "overstretch," even if that feels good to them. They will need to work more on closed pelvis poses and avoid wide-legged poses that put increased stress on the SI joint, such as Baddha Konasana and Upavista Konasana. It is also important to allow the pelvis to move as one unit in forward bends and twists, to avoid excess shearing on the joint. A therapeutic class or program for the SI joint will include postures that keep the hips square and emphasize internal rotation and adduction, as well as a great deal of lower extremity and abdominal strengthening.

SACROILIAC JOINT DYSFUNCTION

Recommendations

- Poses that increase stability in the pelvis
- Closed pelvis poses
- Hip opening
- Standing poses with hips square
- Purna Yoga Low Back Series to decrease pain and traction the sacrum away from the lumbar spine

Contraindications

- Deep twists with pelvis fixed
- Open pelvis poses like Virabahadrasana II (warrior II) and Parsvakonasana (extended side angle stretch) in addition to Baddha Konasana and Supta Baddha Konasana (seated bound angle pose and reclining bound angle pose)
- Because SI joint dysfunction can vary from individual to individual, any pose that causes pain or discomfort should be omitted. For some, forward bends will be more painful, while for others, back bends may cause pain. If you feel worse after a particular practice, pay attention. Usually a strong Vinyasa practice with many repeated movements from forward bends to back bends will aggravate SI joint dysfunction

SI joint sequence

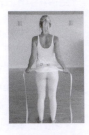

a. Purna Yoga Low Back Series (see Chapter 3)

b. Purna Yoga Hip Opening Series—use blocks for hip internal and external rotation to keep pelvis level (see Chapter 4)

c. SI straps / two belts around pelvis—you can practice with this to decrease SI pain

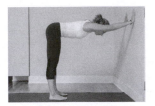

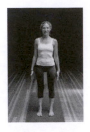

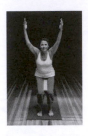

d. Half Uttanasana (half forward fold)

e. Tadasana (mountain pose) with a block between legs

f. Utkatasana (chair pose) with block—emphasize internal rotation of thighs

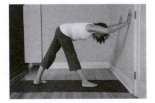

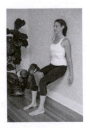

g. Half-Parsvottanasana (half-pyramid pose)

h. Wall squat with block

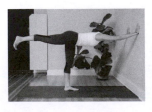

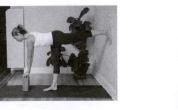

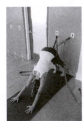

i. Virabhadrasana III (warrior III) with leg on wall, hands on a block

j. Cross straps on yoga wall or door

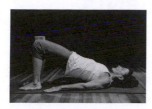

k. Setu Bandha Sarvangasana (bridging) with block between legs; emphasize rotating thighs down toward the floor

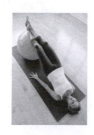

l. Setu Bandha Sarvangasana (advanced bridging) on therapy ball

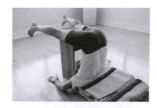

m. Supported Halasana (supported plough pose)

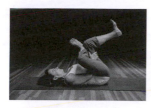

n. Piriformis stretch

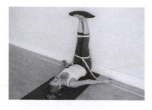

o. Legs up wall with weight

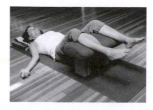

p. Stonehenge Savasana (corpse pose) with support under legs using bolster and two blocks

7. OSTEOPOROSIS/OSTEOPENIA

The World Health Organization (n.d.) reports that osteoporosis is an age-related disease that affects approximately 15 percent of white people in their 50s, and 70 percent of those over 80. It is characterized by a decrease in bone density and an increased risk of fractures, most commonly in the vertebrae, shoulder, wrist, and hip. With osteoporosis there are usually no symptoms until a fracture occurs. Those with osteoporosis tend to develop a kyphosis due to the loss of bone height, and collapse in the anterior portion of the vertebral bodies of the thoracic spine (see Figure 10.7). It is for this reason that forward bending is contraindicated for individuals with osteoporosis. It is also recommended that deep twists be avoided in order to reduce the risk of stress fractures. Loren Fishman (n.d.), in a pilot study using a specific 12-pose yoga protocol, reported on the Sciatica.org website that these safe postures "have improved bone strength and mineral density significantly. DEXA scans were done on volunteers who were then divided into two groups. One group did the yoga, the other did not. After two years the DEXA scans were repeated. They showed a dramatic rise in the bone mineral density of those who practiced yoga. The people that did not do any yoga had an expected modest fall in their bone mineral density."

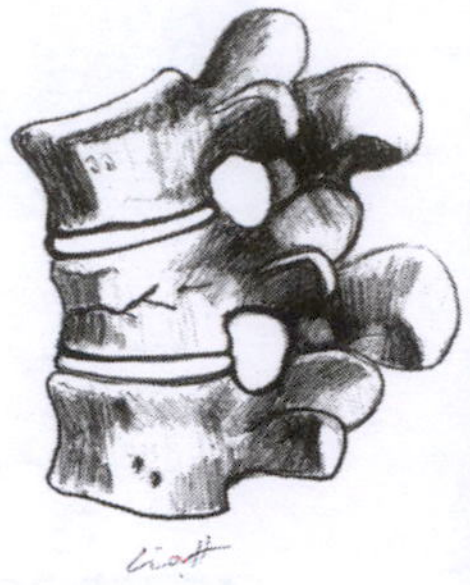

Figure 10.7 Osteoporosis of the thoracic spine

Osteopenia is a precursor to osteoporosis and involves a mild loss of bone density, but not enough to warrant a diagnosis of osteoporosis. Yoga can benefit these individuals greatly and can help reverse or prevent the progress of the disease. There are no contraindications at this stage, other than each person's own pain and physical limitations.

When teaching individuals with osteopenia and osteoporosis, it is important to focus on postures to increase weight bearing on the joints in a safe manner. It is also important to strengthen the back muscles and work on spinal extension postures (modified back bends) to combat the tendency for these individuals to slump forward; these postures include: Bhujangasana (cobra pose); modified Ustrasana (camel pose) with chairs; Setu Bandha Sarvangasana (bridge pose); and Salabhasana (locust pose). Encourage chest and hip opening, as well, to improve posture and normalize the spinal curves. Then teach core strengthening postures such as Uttihita Chaturanga Dandasana (plank pose) (on chair or floor) and Jathara Parivartanasana (revolved abdomen pose), which is a supine twist using the obliques and transversus abdominis to stabilize.

Yoga is most effective in the prevention and healing of osteoporosis in conjunction with changes in lifestyle and nutrition.

OSTEOPOROSIS/OSTEOPENIA

Recommendations

- Weight bearing postures (standing poses and poses with weight on upper body)
- Back bending postures
- Postural exercises
- Hip openers
- Chest openers
- Core stabilization

Contraindications

- Forward bends
- Deep twists (gentle twists are OK)

Osteoporosis/osteopenia sequence

a. Purna Yoga Hip Opening Series (see Chapter 4)

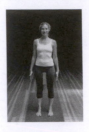

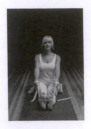

b. Tadasana (mountain pose)— emphasize grounding and pressing all four corners of feet into floor

c. Dandasana (staff pose)— emphasize grounding sitting bones down into floor

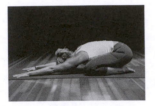

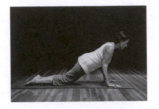

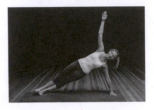

d. Yoga Mudra

e. Phalakasana (plank pose)

f. Vasisthasana (side plank)

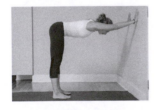

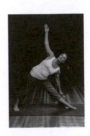

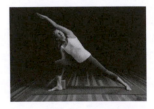

g. Half Uttanasana (half forward fold)

h. Trikonasana (triangle pose)

i. Parsvakonasana (extended side angle stretch)

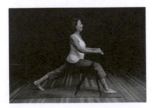

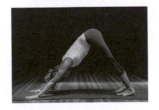

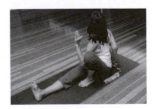

j. Virabhadrasana I (warrior I)

k. Adho Mukha Svanasana (downward-facing dog)

l. Matsyendrasana I (seated spinal twist)—gentle

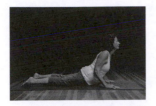

m. Bhujangasana (cobra pose)

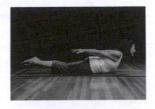

n. Salabhasana (locust pose)

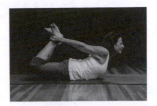

o. Danurasana (bow pose)

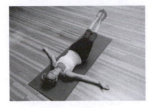

p. Jathara Parivartanasana (revolved abdomen posture)

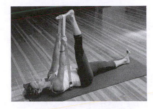

q. Supta Padangusthasana (reclining hand to big toe pose)

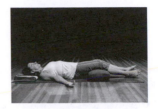

r. Savasana (corpse pose)

8. DISC BULGE/HERNIATION

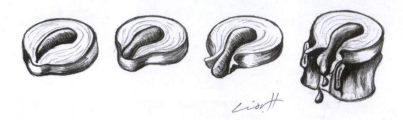

Figure 10.8 Disc bulge/herniation

A bulging disc occurs when the jelly on the inside of the disc protrudes out the back, usually causing compression of one or more nerves and/or the spinal cord. In the case of a disc bulge, the outer membrane of the disc remains intact. In contrast, a disc herniation is when the tough, outer layer of disc cartilage tears and allows the soft inside of the disc to protrude outside of the disc space. While a disc herniation is indeed more dramatic, very often the disc material will dissipate and get reabsorbed into the body, while a bulge can remain in the intervertebral space for a while, causing more pressure on the exiting spinal nerve.

In either case, the main focus of asana practice will be on decompression; therefore, traction techniques and postures to encourage more space in between each vertebra are indicated.

DISC BULGE/HERNIATION

Recommendations

- Purna Yoga Low Back Series
- Spinal traction techniques (no bilateral traction during acute phase)
- Purna Yoga Reversing the Aging of the Spine Series (as tolerated; not in acute stage)
- Purna Yoga Hip Opening Series
- Piriformis stretches
- Psoas openers
- Standing poses with emphasis on length in spine
- Core strengthening in neutral

Contraindications

- No forward bends
- No deep twists

Disc bulge/herniation sequence (not acute phase)

a. Purna Yoga Low Back Series (see Chapter 3)

b. Purna Yoga Hip Opening Series (see Chapter 4)

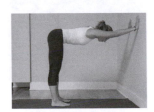

c. Supported lunge

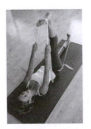

d. Supta Padangusthasana (reclining hand to big toe pose) with two belts

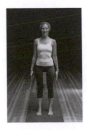

e. Tadasana (mountain pose) with block between legs

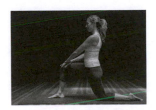

f. Half-Uttanasana (half forward fold)

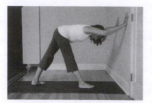

g. Half-Parsvottanasana
(half-pyramid pose)

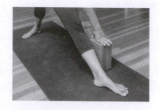

h. Trikonasana (triangle pose) with
front foot in external rotation

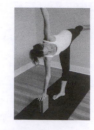

i. Ardha Chandrasana (half-
moon pose) with front foot
in external rotation

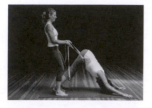

j. Adho Mukha Svanasana
(downward-facing dog) with
wall rope or partner for traction

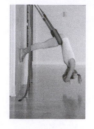

k. Hanging traction on wall rope

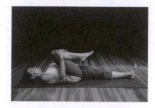

l. Half-Apanasana (single
knee to chest)

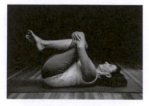

m. Apanasana (double
knees to chest)

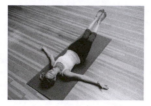

n. Gentle Jathara Parivartanasana
(revolved abdomen pose)
with knees bent

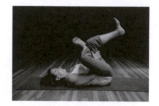

o. Supine piriformis stretch
(pigeon pose)

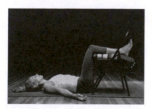

p. Savasana (corpse pose)
with bolster under knees
or legs on chair

9. SCIATICA VS. PIRIFORMIS SYNDROME

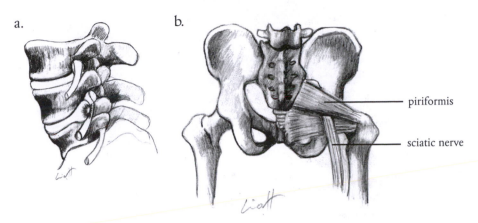

Figure 10.9 a. True sciatica (nerve is pinched in lumbar spine); b. piriformis syndrome (nerve is pinched behind the pirifromis muscles)

Sciatica is not a diagnosis, but rather is a set of symptoms, which can include pain in the lower back, buttock, or parts of the leg or foot. Sciatica may be caused by compression or irritation of one of the five spinal nerve roots in the lower lumbar spine (L1–5) that join to create each sciatic nerve. This is called "true sciatica" because the compression is in the lumbar spine, where the origin of the sciatic nerve is found.

Piriformis syndrome is a disorder that occurs when the piriformis muscle deep in the buttocks compresses or irritates the sciatic nerve, resulting in pain, tingling, or numbness in the lower back, leg, and foot. This is called "false sciatica," as it mimics all of the symptoms of true sciatica, but the problem is due to tightness or inflammation in the piriformis muscle. Piriformis syndrome is suspected as a possible diagnosis when there is no clear spinal cause (i.e. herniated disc) for sciatica.

It is easier to treat piriformis syndrome than true sciatica, as the treatment entails decreasing inflammation and stretching of the piriformis muscle as well as the surrounding hip musculature. Treatment for true sciatica that originates in the lumbar spine requires decompression, as above in the sequence for disc bulge/herniation.

Sciatica recommendations and sequence

Same as the disc bulge/herniation recomendations and sequence above.

Piriformis Syndrome

Recommendations

- Purna Yoga Hip Opening Series —with a focus on internal rotation; skip external rotation
- Piriformis stretches
- Tadasana (mountain pose) with block between the legs to turn off the external hip rotators
- Poses that emphasize internal rotation of the hips, i.e. closed pelvis poses
- Psoas openers
- Pigeon toe walking

Contraindications

- No forward bends if they increase symptoms
- No postures that activate the external rotators of the hip

Piriformis syndrome sequence

a. Purna Yoga Hip Opening Series (see Chapter 4)

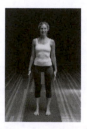

b. Tadasana (mountain pose) with block—emphasis on internal rotation of thighs, decreasing external rotation in hips, relaxing buttocks

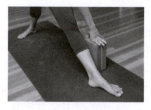

c. Trikonasana (triangle pose) with foot in external rotation

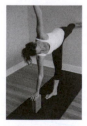

d. Ardha Chandrasana (half-moon pose) with foot in external rotation

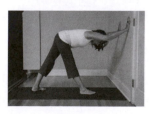

e. Half-Parsvattanasana (half-pyramid pose)

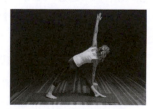

f. Parivrtta Trikonasana (revolving triangle pose)

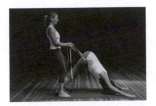

g. *Adho Mukha Svanasana (downward-facing dog) on wall ropes or with partners for traction*

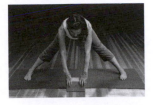

h. *Prasarita Padottanasana (wide-legged forward fold)*

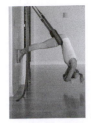

i. *Hanging traction on wall ropes*

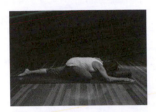

j. *Supported pigeon pose on bolster*

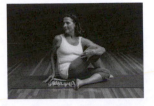

k. *Ardha Matsyendrasana (half lord of the fishes pose)*

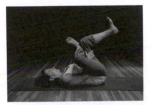

l. *Supine piriformis stretch*

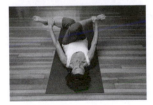

m. *Supine outer hip stretch (cross legs at knees, holding onto ankles)*

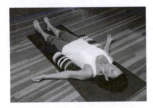

n. *Savasana (corpse pose) with blankets on outer hips to decrease external rotation in hips*

These targeted sequences for specific conditions should be accompanied by various breathing techniques, affirmations, meditations, and all the other elements of a balanced yoga practice in order to address all layers (koshas) of each individual. Incorporating all the elements in yoga—not just the physical or *annamaya kosha*—is integral in helping the client to release stress and tension, and move more deeply into self-exploration and from that into expanded awareness, to find the attitude and courage to support a healing process that will serve them for a lifetime.

References

Berceli, D. (2008) *The Revolutionary Trauma Release Process: Transcend Your Toughest Times*. Vancouver: Namaste Publishing.

Bogduk, N. (2000) 'What's in a name? The labelling of back pain.' *The Medical Journal of Australia 173*, 8, 400–401.

Borenstein, D.G., O'Mara, J.W. Jr., Boden, S.D., *et al.* (2001) 'The value of magnetic resonance imaging of the lumbar spine to predict low-back pain in asymptomatic subjects: a seven-year follow-up study.' *Journal of Bone and Joint Surgery 83*, 1306–1311. Available at www.ncbi.nlm.nih.gov/pubmed/11568190, accessed on 17 March 2016.

Brach, T. (2013) *True Refuge: Finding Peace and Freedom in Your Own Awakened Heart*. New York: Bantam Books.

Brourman, S. (1998/2007) *Walk Yourself Well: Eliminate Back Pain, Neck, Shoulder, Knee, Hip and Other Structural Pain Forever—Without Surgery or Drugs*. Santa Monica, CA: Author.

Davis, K.G., Marras, W.S., Heaney, C.A., Waters, T.R. and Gupta, P. (2002) 'The impact of mental processing and pacing on spinal loading: 2002 Volvo Award in Biomechanics.' *Spine 27*, 23, 2645–2653.

Deyo, R.A. and Weinstein, J.N. (2001) 'Low back pain.' *The New England Journal of Medicine 344*, 363–370. doi:10.1056/NEJM200102013440508.

Ellis. J. (2006) 'Lumbo-pelvic integration: an integrated approach to the management of somatic dysfunction of the lumbar spine and pelvic girdle regions.' *LPI Course Workbook*. New York: Integrative Manual Therapy Solutions.

Fishman, L.M. (n.d.) *A Dozen Poses vs. Osteoarthritis*. Available at www.sciatica.org/yoga/12poses.html, accessed on 12 July 2015.

Fishman, L.M., Groessl, E.J., and Sherman, K.J. (2014) 'Serial case reporting yoga for idiopathic and degenerative scoliosis.' *Global Advances in Health and Medicine 3*, 5, 16–21. Available at www.gahmj.com/doi/full/10.7453/gahmj.2013.064, accessed on 8 February 2015.

Haig, A.J., Tong, H.C., Yamakawa, K.S., *et al.* (2006) 'Spinal stenosis, back pain, or no symptoms at all? A masked study comparing radiologic and electrodiagnostic diagnoses to the clinical impression.' *Archives of Physical Medicine and Rehabilitation 87*, 7, 897–903. Available at www.ncbi.nlm.nih.gov/pubmed/16813774, accessed on 17 March 2016.

Hauser, R.A., Dolan, E.E., Phillips, H.J., Newlan, A.C., Moore, R.E., and Woldin, B.A. (2013) 'Ligament injury and healing: a review of current clinical diagnostics and therapeutics.' *The Open Rehabilitation Journal 6*, 1–20.

Hides, J., Stanton, W., Mendis, M.D., and Sexton, M. (2011) 'The relationship of transversus abdominis and lumbar multifidus clinical muscle tests in patients with chronic low back pain.' *Manual Therapy 16*, 6, 573–577. doi:10.1016/j.math.2011.05.007.

Hodges, P.W. and Richardson, C.A. (1996) 'Inefficient muscular stabilization of the lumbar spine associated with low back pain: a motor control evaluation of transversus abdominis.' *Spine 21*, 22, 2640–2650.

International Infopage for Ashtanga Yoga: Yoga Sutras of Patanjali. Available at www.ashtangayoga.info/source-texts/yoga-sutra-patanjali/chapter-1, accessed on 26 May 2015.

Hoge, K.M., Ryan, E.D., Costa, P.B., et al. (2010) 'Gender differences in musculotendinous stiffness and range of motion after an acute bout of stretching.' *Journal of Strength and Conditioning Research 24*, 10, 2618–2626.

Iyengar, B.K.S. (2005) *Light on Life*. London: Pan Macmillan.

Jensen, M.J., Brant-Zawadzki, M.N., Obuchowski, N., Modic, M.T., Malkasian, D. and Ross, J.S. (1994). 'Magnetic resonance imaging of the lumbar spine in people without back pain.' *The New England Journal of Medicine 331*, 2, 6–73.

Kleinman, D.M. (2009) 'Knee laxity tied to menstrual cycle.' *Musculoskeletal Rep*, quoted by R.A Hauser., E.E. Dolan, H.J. Phillips, A.C. Newlan, R.E. Moore and B.A. Woldin (2013) 'Ligament injury and healing: a review of current clinical diagnostics and therapeutics.' *The Open Rehabilitation Journal 6*, 1–20, 2.

Knutson, G.A. (2005) 'Anatomic and functional leg-length inequality: a review and recommendation for clinical decision-making. Part I, anatomic leg-length inequality: prevalence, magnitude, effects and clinical significance.' *Chiropractic and Osteopathy 13*, 11. Available at www.ncbi.nlm.nih.gov/pmc/articles/PMC1232860, accessed on 17 March 2016.

Koch, L. (1981/2012) *The Psoas Book: A Guide to the Iliopsoas Muscle and Its Effect on the Body, Mind, and Emotions*. Felton, CA: Guinea Pig Publications.

Koch, L. (2011) *Pulling It All Together: Psoas, Fear and Core Strength*. Available at www.pilatesunion.com/news/24, accessed on 17 March 2016.

Kos, J., Hert, J., and Sevcík, P. (2002) 'Meniscoids of the intervertebral joints.' *Acta Chir Orthop Traumatol Cech 69*, 3, 149–157.

Krentzman, R. (in press) *Scoliosis, Yoga Therapy and the Art of Letting Go*. London: Singing Dragon.

Kumar, A., Kumar, S., and Kumar, R. (2012) 'Effectiveness of pelvic floor muscle exercise and bladder training in stress urinary incontinence and low back discomfort—a case study.' *Yoga and Physical Therapy 2*, 5, 1–3.

Lasater, J.H. (2005) *Yoga Abs: Moving from your Core*. Berkeley, CA: Rodmell Press.

Lasater, J.H. (2009) *Yoga Body: Anatomy, Kinesiology, and Yoga*. Berkeley, CA: Rodmell Press.

Lederman, E. (2007) 'The myth of core stability.' *CPDO Online Journal*, 1–17. Available at www.cpdo.net, accessed on 17 March 2016.

Levine, P.A. (1997) *Waking the Tiger*. Berkeley, CA: North Atlantic Books.

McLean, A. (2015) 'Issues of the pelvic floor: a current literature review.' Unpublished final paper, Yoga for a Happy Back Mentorship Program.

Mens, J., Hoek van Dijke, G.A., Pool-Goedzwaard, A., van der Hulst, V., and Stam, H. (2006) 'Possible harmful effects of high intra-abdominal pressure on the pelvic girdle.' *Journal of Biomechanics 39*, 4, 627–635.

naturalheightgrowth.com (2014) *Can Twisting Increase Vetebral Disc Length?* Available at www.naturalheightgrowth.com/2014/02/06/can-twisting-increase-vertebral-disc-length, accessed on 28 March 2015.

Palkhivala, A. (2008a) *Fire of Love*. Bellevue, WA: The Innerworks Company.

Palkhivala, A. (2008b) *Purna Yoga 200 Hour Teacher Training Manual*. Bellevue, WA: Alive and Shine Center. *Purna Yoga™ founded by Aadil Palkhivala and Savitri*.

Pascual-Leone, A., Freitas, C., Oberman, L., *et al.* (2011) 'Characterizing brain cortical plasticity and network dynamics across the age-span in health and disease with TMS-EEG and TMS-fMRI.' *Brain Topography 24*, 302–315.

Prosko, S. (2014) 'The truth about back pain: a biopsychosocial approach to treatment.' *Yoga Therapy Today*, Summer 2014, 28–34.

Ryanno, T. (2007) 'Kinematics of the lumbar spine in trunk rotation: in vivo three-dimensional analysis using magnetic resonance imaging.' *European Spine Journal 16*, 11, 1867–1874.

Sapsford, R. (2004) 'Rehabilitation of pelvic floor muscles utilizing trunk stabilization.' *Manual Therapy 9*, 3–12.

Sarno, J. (1991) *Healing Back Pain*. New York: Warner Books/Hachette Book Group.

Satchidananda, Sri Swami, translator (1978/2010) *The Yoga Sutras of Patanjali*. Buckingham, VA: Integral Yoga Publications.

Savitri (2016) *Heartfull™ Meditation Snack Techniques*. Bellevue, WA. *Heartfull™ Meditation, Philosophy & Lifestyle, created by Savitri*.

Scerpella, T.A., Stayer, T.J., Makhuli, B.Z. (2005) 'Ligamentous laxity and non-contact anterior cruciate ligament tear: a gender-based comparison.' *Orthopedics 28*, 656.

Sivananda, Swami (1993) *The Ten Upanishads*. Himalayas, India: The Divine Life Society.

Stevenson, J.C. (2012) *Low Back Pain's Missing Link*. The Orthopaedic Institute. Available at www.toi-health.com/low-back-pains-missing-link-diagnosing-the-sacroiliac-joint.aspx, accessed on 28 December 2014.

Vivekananda, Swami (2003) *Raja Yoga*. New York: Celephaïs Press.

WebMD (n.d.) *Scoliosis: What is Scoliosis?* Available at www.webmd.com/osteoarthritis/guide/arthritis-scoliosis, accessed on 20 July 2015.

World Health Organization (n.d.) Osteoporosis. Available at www.who.int/chp/topics/rheumatic/en, accessed 14 July 2015.

Index

legs up the wall pose
    for sacroiliac joint dysfunction 143
Levine, Peter 207, 208
Light on Life (Iyengar) 55

Makhuli, B.Z. 28
March Test 66–7, 78
McLean, A. 187
Medical Journal of Australia 47
meditation
    Heartfull™ meditation
        techniques 223–5
    starting 221–3
Mens, J. 179
mountain pose
    for back pain relief 98
    for hip strengthening 123, 125
    for sacroiliac joint dysfunction 139–40
    and spinal curvature 36, 37, 39
    and standing poses 246
movement dysfunction
    description of 55–6
    evaluation of 59–78
    in practice of yoga 56–7
    and structural dysfunction 53–8
multifidus muscle 184–5

Nadi Shodhana
    as preparation for Pranayama 219
Navasana
    connecting to the core 188–92
neuromuscular scan 66
New England Journal of Medicine 47
Niyamas 253–4

Open Rehabilitation Journal 27
Orthopedics 27
osteopenia
    poses for 278–81
osteoporosis
    poses for278–81

Padangusthasana 192
pain
    balance between stability and
        mobility 27, 29–33
    changing story of 21–4
    finding true self 41–2

as gateway 22–4
healing 42
layers of 25–7
maintaining spine curvature 34–9
movement with 39–41
principles for healing 20–45
source of 58–9
and structural vs. movement
    dysfunction 54–8
Palkhivala, Aadil 16, 200
    attitude to pain 24
    on illness 20
    inspiration from 254
    and lower back 81
    and Purna Yoga Hip Opening
        Series 94, 115
    and spinal curvature 48
    on teaching yoga 230, 258
    and traction techniques 162
    on yoga 177, 211–12
Parivrtta Supta Padangusthasana
    and hip movement 116
Parsva Supta Padangusthasana
    and hip movement 117
Parsvottanasana
    and hamstring openers 231–2
    for sacroiliac joint 145, 146
Pascual–Leone, A. 222
pelvic floor 186–8
pelvic swing
    as traction technique 161–2
pelvis
    effects on spine 106
Phalakasana
    for strengthening abdominal
        muscles 196–7
piriformis muscle 110
piriformis syndrome
    poses for 285–7
pit of the abdomen 48, 49, 88, 89,
    90, 91, 99, 193, 215, 218, 233
plank pose
    for strengthening abdominal
        muscles 196–7
plow pose
    for sacroiliac joint dysfunction 142–3